I LOVE ME MORE THAN SUGAR

THE WHY AND HOW OF 30 DAYS SUGAR FREE

BARRY FRIEDMAN

"This fast moving, factual, life-changing book gives you great ideas on how to improve your diet, lose weight, increase energy, and be healthier for the rest of your life." —*Brian Tracy*
#1 Bestselling Author, The Power of Self-Confidence

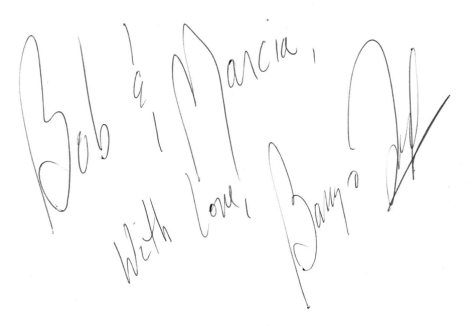

Bob & Marcia,
With love, Barry

To my son Zed who lights up my life and inspires me to live forever.
You bring more sweetness into my life than sugar ever could.

And to my wife Annie. You are my greatest mirror and that reflection
has formed who I am today. Believing in me since 1986... I'm sure
I would have left me by now.

Contents

Taste • Living and Eating with Others • Mindset Tips • The Most Important Meal of the Day • What About Lunch? • Dinner: Graze, Don't Gorge • Snacks • Big Events • Falling off the Wagon

PART III: THE CHALLENGE

Introduction

How I Got Here

I've been preparing to write this book for 51-years. And while that might sound like one wicked case of writer's block, I can assure you that's not the case. My preparation probably has a lot in common with your preparation for reading this book: we were both raised on diets that were inspired by industrial advances during the Baby Boomer generation.

Fed baby formula where two of the first three ingredients are sugar? Yep.

Bribed to behave, listen up, or act a certain way with the promise of a treat? Oh, yeah!

Punished by having dessert, candy, or soda withheld? Standard issue in my family.

Shown love with a birthday cake or a box of Valentine's Day candy? Given an ice cream sundae or fresh chocolate chip cookie when feeling down? Don't mind if I do.

Over-indulgence with sugar has been a part of my life since the moment I was conceived. From what I heard, there might even have been an onslaught of sugar that led up to the act itself.

But I digress.

I was 49 years old on February 28, 2012. It was a leap year and my son, then 9 years old, was intrigued with the idea of such a day. Being very involved in his education, I try not to miss the opportunity for a teaching moment so I jumped into action.

"Leap Day, historically, is where you leap right over something you would normally do," I said, trying to make my explanation sound plausible. "A habit or ritual that you do every other day of the year is leaped over on Leap Day."

I actually didn't think it was such a bad idea.

"What are you going to leap over, Daddy?" he asked.

It was an unseasonably warm February afternoon and I drove home from the yogurt shop after polishing off a cup of frozen dessert with all the toppings. My stomach was turning flips trying to reconcile gummy bears and mini-chocolate peanut butter cups as my body set in for the post-sugar crash.

"Sugar. I'm going to skip sugar for the day."

As he extended his tongue toward the bottom of his cup, he assured me that he would not be joining me in that leap. Instead, he announced he'd leap the act of picking his nose. We all have our battles.

I don't know about you, but when I say something to my son, it cures like that quick-dry cement. There has to be a jackhammer-sized reason for me to go back on it and even then, it's not easy. I know that everything I do shows up on an IMAX-sized screen in his mind and will cumulatively guide him toward how he shows up in the world.

Cut to me, February 29th, 2012, heading into the kitchen for breakfast. I had given the sugar free day a bit of thought the night before, but now I was facing reality. The cupboard held nothing edible to someone with a mission so noble as mine. I was not going to let anything get in the way of me spending the day without processed or refined sugar. The fridge had a 1/2 gallon of milk and I had an idea: oatmeal with almonds, raisins, and milk. Look at me—a sugar free breakfast and feeling like I had this thing whipped.

I took one bite and froze. It tasted like cardboard. Wet, mushy, cardboard. My tongue tried to push it out past my clenched teeth while my throat refused to yield and allow passage. This was going to be a very long day.

Where was the heaping tablespoon of brown sugar that made this taste more like the oatmeal I was used to eating and less like mortar?

I saw a banana on the counter and jumped up to cut it into small pieces. It was a race against time as I could almost hear the cereal hardening. Putting some of my weight behind the spoon, I was able to work the banana pieces into the mix. It was a vast improvement and in six minutes I finished the bowl. My palms started sweating as I contemplated what I would eat for the rest of the day. I told myself that tomorrow I would add extra sugar to everything I ate just to make up for today.

I navigated the remainder of the day with careful execution. Lunch was simple: tuna and celery with some potato chips. For dinner we had a chicken stir fry and I skipped the sauce because the third ingredient was "evaporated cane juice" and I knew what that meant.

I didn't want to be awake for the mandatory 10 p.m. refrigerator raid that was as much a part of my night as hating myself for doing it. That pointless feast was an agreement between me and my emotional shortcomings and I didn't want to show up empty-handed with my sad story about no sugar. I was in bed at 8:15 p.m.

As I lay there, I noticed a few things that I liked. I hadn't felt a sugar crash all day. My stomach was calm and easy which was unusual for me. At my normal bedtime of 11:00 p.m., there was usually something noisy happening down there. I had a smile on my face and that really got me thinking... maybe I could do 30 days of this?

And there it was—that one thought had passed through my cranium and I knew I wasn't going to sell myself short. I called my wife into the room (I wasn't going to get up and walk past the fridge—it was mad at me!) and made the commitment. After 25 years together, she knows my brain is like a pit bull with a mailman. Once the teeth are in, it's very difficult to unlock the jaw.

I'll spare you the non-drama of days two and three, instead, providing you a ringside seat to the raging agony of Day 4. It'll make for a better read and impress upon you the level of my (and possibly your) addiction to the white stuff.

Day 4 started out innocently enough. Some part of my creative, improvisational right brain told its more analytical left-sided neighbor that we had done amazingly well for the past three days and we should have a bit of sugar that morning. Just some cereal—nothing bad. I felt the idea bounce off the left lobe and smack the right hemisphere square in the synapses. I shut down, feeling edgy, shaky, and emotional. By noon I was hungry, crying, and desperately needed to climb out of my own skin.

My wife offered me a massage and I couldn't lie still enough to have it make sense. I was in full detox mode and the various systems of my body were working together to get me to crumble. This was exactly what I imagined happens to people who go cold turkey off of heroin or speed. This is not where I imagined steering clear of cookies and ice cream would land me. I was cranky, uncomfortable—and fascinated.

I recommitted to the 30 days right then and there and I felt some of the fight inside of me fall over and die. By 3:00 p.m. that day I was drinking a ton of water, exercising, and recovering from the battle that I hosted on my own internal Lexington and Concord. The habits of the past five decades had come face to face with the desires of my next incarnation and I was a heap of cells just holding on.

Why did I pull out Day 4 at this point in the book while we are just getting to know each other? It has to do with the authenticity of this experience and life change that you might be contemplating. You see, there is nothing about the early days of going sugar free that are glamorous. While nothing like Day 4 ever happened again, the rest of those 30 days were nothing to brag about. I didn't make any new friends, win the father-of-the-month award, or endear myself to my wife.

Change takes change and it would have been a hundred times easier to stay exactly where I was. Since quitting sugar I have lost 15% of my body weight, my skin looks better than it did when I was 30, I'm wearing the same size pants I wore in high school (32" waist!), and I have more energy than ever before. Without that one decision, I would be less of a man, husband, and father. If I folded on Day 4, there would be thousands of people around the world who would still be suffering from excess weight, poor sleep, anxiety, high blood pressure, depression, skin problems, and poor focus. Those are just some of the changes that have been reported from those I have coached through 30, 60, 90 days, and/or a commitment to a lifetime of sugar free eating.

Who Am I?

Maybe you've seen me on TV (either talking about the sugar free lifestyle or in my role as a four-time World Juggling Champion—more on that later), been in one of my online programs, or perhaps this is the first time you've ever heard the names Barry and Friedman in succession. The fact is that the only reason we are spending this time together right now is because I stood in the fire on Day 4 and refused to let the old ways kill my dream of living healthier and showing up bigger for my son, my wife, myself, and the world.

I've been a professional coach since 2009. Thousands of people around the world have been guided by my writing, teaching, lecturing, or one-on-one coaching in the fields of business and/or sugar free living. I also have an active leadership and coaching role in the Boys to Men Mentoring Network for youth ages 9–17.

While I've studied piles of research and talked at length with nutritionists, doctors, and health experts, I'm proud to be a non-scientific representative for what's possible when we make conscious choices about what we put into our bodies. I didn't get this life change approved by my doctor. I don't study calorie charts or measure my calories. I eat real foods without any refined or processed sugar and I never miss a chance to inspire others who are ready to take a look at who they want to be in relation to sugar.

In this book, I dispel a number of myths about food and health. I show you exactly what it takes to go from where you are now to where you want to be. And, more than anything else, I promise to take you to the place where—perhaps for the only time in your entire life—you will be far enough away from sugar's intoxicating spell to make an honest choice about what part it will play in the rest of your life.

How to Use This Book

Within these pages, I offer a 30 day challenge in which the goal is to get you through those 30 days without eating processed or refined sugar. That is the expectation. This is not a plan specifically for reducing weight. That said, throughout the 30 days you'll learn to set measurable and realistic goals which can certainly include the goal of weight loss. You'll be challenged to add exercise into your daily routine. Along with eating sugar free, this typically results in weight loss.

To get the most out of this book, you will be asked to examine personal experiences and provide feedback through journaling and exercises to anchor your experience.

Additional support and information is available through the companion web site to this book. It is a free resource to my readers and you are encouraged to use it as you read this book. I'll occasionally refer to the Member Area and you can find it by visiting this link: http://ILoveMeMoreThanSugar.com

The first time you visit, you will be asked to register a username and password. You will then have free, lifetime access to the Member Area. Store or write down your username and password as you'll need it for future visits.

Ready to Go?

Welcome to a world where the possibility exists that for a week you'll feel better on Wednesday than you did on Tuesday; for a year where you'll be stronger in June than you were in January. If you decide that you do indeed love yourself more than sugar, a whole new paradigm in life awaits you. You'll have passage into a world where the old rules don't apply, empowering you to make choices that support the biggest and brightest version of yourself—easily and automatically.

Just by living that life, you will hold up a mirror of possibility for your friends and family.

Barry Friedman
December 1, 2014

PART I: WHY

CHAPTER 1
Your Big Why

Let's be clear right up front—there is almost no chance of you being talked into doing this. This isn't like picking up trash on the side of the highway or going to traffic school to get a ticket off your record—those are easy because they are court ordered.

No, the motivation for giving yourself 30 Days Sugar Free has to come from within. That's the only place that houses the power that you'll need to keep going. Honestly, during those early days when it's late at night and both a cookie and your mouth are dying to meet, it's an inner power that will keep your hand from connecting the two.

Sure, external forces can help. If a doctor with a wall full of degrees proving she's smarter than you told you to go cold-turkey off of all processed and refined sugars, it would be easier.

The Inner Game of 30 Days Sugar Free

This is the part of the book where I should be telling you all the good reasons to treat your body to 30 Days Sugar Free. Maybe paint the picture of how healthy, thin, and calm you'll feel when your body isn't freaking out from a dose of high fructose corn syrup, evaporated cane juice, dextrose, or any of the other 50+ shades of sugar.

The truth is—this is an internal game. Success or failure is up to you!

This isn't a governmental or bureaucratic problem. It's a personal one. Governments and other bureaucracies seem to be overly wrapped in red tape and operate on a never-ending time line. You and I, on the other hand, get moment to moment feedback on how we're feeling and have a much more tangible shelf life.

In the 2014 documentary film *Fed Up*, the filmmakers uncover more than a dozen culprits that sell, advertise, produce, tout, and encourage behaviors and consumption that are making our children fat, sick, and tired. They clearly state that a child today is part of the first generation in history expected to lead a shorter life than his or her parents. Read that again and breathe it in. This is the first generation in history expected to lead a shorter life than his or her parents. Definitively a heavy dose of downer—and an important message to hear.

In the film, there is a whole lot of finger pointing at big, faceless entities including medicine, food manufactures, and every political office from Mayor to President. I am concerned most with the connection between one's own hand and mouth. While we could debate the economic and cultural influences surrounding sugar, it all comes down to what you decide to put into your mouth. That is the moment of choice. Yes, it's horrible and sad that kids are exposed to hours of ads for foods that will take them directly from innocence to being a statistic. The more we allow media to educate our children, the less say we have in how they eat, think, or behave. Our precious children are just doing what they are taught.

Our addiction to sugar isn't going to be solved by someone else and delivered in a neat package, pill, or protocol. It's not going to be solved by parents who eat crap while telling their kids to eat healthy; by adults that text while driving yet tell the kids to stop being addicted to their media devices; or by those who are out of shape and demand that their kids get outside and exercise. Most important for this generation of kids is what's in the home.

Kids tend to emulate what they see and how they are brought up. Every one of the four kids portrayed in *Fed Up* had either one or two overweight parents. The problem is generational and change takes change. Hard, difficult change. Hero's Journey work. We'll talk about that later.

You Inspire People in Your Life

You know you're being watched, don't you? I'm not talking about a creepy or illegal way. I mean you are being watched by the people in your life. They notice what you are doing, not doing, eating, wearing, reading, and saying. This includes people you know and those you happen upon.

Your friends, co-workers, or the person sitting next to you on an airplane are all using you as one of the factors in what they do, don't do, eat, wear, read, and say.

Not to pour a gallon of pressure over your head, but if you have kids, all of this is amplified a hundred times. For the formative years of their life they are acutely tuned into all things "you". They know the version of you that doesn't wear the work, social, or superhero mask required in other areas of your life. They aren't burdened with any of the responsibilities or distractions that get in the way of their full-time study of you.

What does this have to do with why you might want to do 30 Days Sugar Free?

Fact: 43% of children and 70% of adults in America are overweight or obese.

The children are watching. A little girl sees her mom carrying an extra 50 lbs and she tells herself it's perfectly fine while she dips her donut into a glass of soda. Is mom programming her daughter for a vibrant life or one plagued with disease?

A boy sees his dad limping, suffering with lower back pain, and sporting a gut that hangs over the top of his jeans. The boy knows he can't run or bike with his dad and that's just the way it is. Instead of being physical together, they sit, watch TV, eat sugary treats, and become more alike. I'm happy that they find common ground, yet I'll forever believe there are possibilities that promote a healthier connection.

According to the Center for Disease Control, kids who are overweight or obese at age 10 are five times more likely to be overweight or obese as adults. Obese kids are more likely to have pre-diabetes and have a greater risk of bone and joint problems, sleep apnea, and social/psychological problems such as stigmatization and poor self-esteem. It's a situation that rarely turns around as children age.

The Oldest Part of Our Brain

In the 50's, doctor and researcher, Paul McClean, discovered that the brain has three main parts.

The first and oldest part of our brain is the "R-Complex," also known as the Reptilian Brain, or as I prefer: *The Lizard Brain.*

Some of the traits associated with it are: protection, aggression, dominance, obsessiveness, compulsiveness, fear, and greed. It drives fundamental survival needs. If you are like most people in our modern society, the use of sugar is viewed by this part of the brain as a survival need. Take it away and someone is going to pay.

If you think you would be worse off at the conclusion of 30 Days Sugar Free, please slap yourself silly. That belief is being heavily influenced by that Lizard Brain. Its job is to protect you from change.

This part of our brain usually has at least one hand on the steering wheel of your life. It's got speed-dial access to your control center and delivers HD quality messages:

"You could never do that."

"You look and feel fine just the way you are."

"What fun could you possibly have going 30 Days Sugar Free?"

It's the part of the brain that—more than anything else—wants everything to stay the same. Don't rock the boat, baby.

What exactly is the voice that will seductively whisper sweet messages to you? It's that part of you that insists on a status quo; a part of you that fears and resists change and has no interest in the dreams you have of feeling better, looking younger, or being healthier. That voice has its own agenda—and it's not a complicated one:

"Protect Barry from danger by keeping things exactly the same. Day after day. Year after year. All that talk about sugar free is scary and dangerous and I must keep Barry away from it. Have a cookie. Have another. There, isn't that better?"

Ancient and set in its ways. Fight or flight.

The yes/no battle that's going on inside your brain is old Lizard's favorite Olympic event. Wiggle room is his playground because he'll dredge up an old belief, memory, or situation that will hurt less if you will agree to eat something sweet. Now!

That part of your brain is fed by you giving in—sugar, TV, sex, drugs—or just about anything else that will deliver a temporary dopamine surge and make sure you stay right where you are. On the other hand, each time you say "No," it loses some control! The Lizard Brain voice gets softer and less convincing. You build credits by standing strong; by being with the sadness, fear, shame, guilt, or anger; by blessing the body with what it really needs—good nutrition, water, exercise, deep breathing, and a calm mind.

At some point, it will be a wimpy, withering whisper—almost laughable. You'll be far enough away from the JUST DO IT addiction to make conscious choices that support the healthiest version of yourself. Hang on to hear it, will you?

30 Days Sugar Free. Why? Why Not?

Why should you do this challenge?

Maybe it's because you came across this book and for some reason, you're reading it. You might be curious about your addiction to foods rich in processed and refined sugar.

Addiction? Me? I can hear the indignation and the resignation—yes, that's right, a bit of both.

If you eat sugar, you are probably more addicted than you think. Sugar isn't designed for satisfaction or completion.

Let's go back to the brain. The moment sugar hits the taste buds on your tongue, a celebration in the brain's reward system is triggered. This part of the cerebral cortex is the hub of a complex network of electrochemical actions and reactions that answers one single question: should I do that again?

Right up until the moment when another condition (stomach ache, guilt, shame, toothache, embarrassment, etc) trumps—the answer is always a resounding "Yes"!

There's not anything wrong with you, my friend. Don't crawl into the rabbit hole of thinking this is a character flaw. It's just chemistry at work. We are the test tubes and this experiment is repeated billions of times each day. Always the same. Always fair.

Perhaps you are reading this and wondering if the amount of sugar you eat is responsible for why you often feel sick, tired, or achy. It's quite possible—dare I say, even probable.

Ideally, sugar is delivered to our system in small doses wrapped up in fiber. Example: an apple. Our bodies can efficiently convert this into energy that feeds our cells and the fiber allows it a slow, responsible release into the system. The apple gives us sustained energy over a period of time. Just what the doctor ordered!

Much of today's sugar, however, is delivered by the boatload in forms that are cooked down, overly concentrated, processed and reprocessed, and void of fiber.

We haven't evolved quickly enough to stand a chance against this quantity of sugar and rate of absorption. With sugar in everything from toothpaste to table salt, most people live in a constant state of processing some form of sugar. While the human body does the best it can, it's losing the battle. Causalities include an increased susceptibility to weight gain, insomnia, anxiety, tooth decay, gout, liver disease, moodiness, high blood pressure, diabetes, and acne. It also delivers a devastating blow to the adrenal glands, cultivates insulin resistance, and taxes your cardiovascular system. There is research showing that cancer cells are happiest when feeding on sugar.

So, could refined sugar be what's making you sick, tired, and achy? Straight from the category of anecdotal medicine—heck yes! Personally, I haven't had a cold, flu, sore throat, or fever since the day I quit eating processed or refined sugar. Even if it's not making you sick, it sure isn't keeping you healthy.

Those in charge of food manufacturing are answering to shareholders who demand bigger returns. They are supported by clever marketing teams who conjure up a leprechaun to boast health benefits of Lucky Charms cereal, words like 'Amino Sweet' to disguise chemical sweeteners, and pictures of strong athletes who would look very different if they actually ate what they endorsed.

Finally, you might be reading this book because you are listening to what the Hawaiians call the na'au. In English that translates to Gut Intelligence. It's your ancient, instinctual wisdom telling you to listen up. It's the intelligence that kept us alive before the industrial revolution but has yielded its power to the more verbal, logical, and modern forms of thinking.

Why the Lizard Usually Wins

So why aren't we driven by the na'au? The logical mind uses verbs and nouns. It has the ability to reiterate and reference; plot and execute. It is heavily influenced by a jumble of pressures which couldn't be any less interesting to the Gut Intelligence. These include:

- Marketing
- Social media
- Recommendations
- Memory
- Propaganda
- Indecision
- Analysis paralysis
- Pretty pictures on the package
- Coupons!

The Gut Intelligence, on the other hand, simply issues its opinion and returns to its post, standing guard for the next opportunity it has to keep you alive. That's exactly what our intuition, or Gut Intelligence, has done since the first caveman turned and ran from a lion. Input, then back to ready position.

In a world where important decisions are often made by the number of LIKES on Facebook, the voting power of the na'au has been reduced to that of a cable station intern in Albuquerque. That 19-year old might have dreams of being the anchorman of NBC news one day, but for now he's best off making sure there are enough rubber bands in the supply cabinet.

Can you feel the paradox between the Lizard Brain and the Gut Intelligence? Both want what they believe to be best for the host, however, in many instances the desired actions are contradictory. Making change in your life will often require you to mute the Lizard Brain long enough and often enough for it to feel safe. Change takes change.

While the Lizard Brain is old, so is our Gut Intelligence. It will never leave our DNA. It's just too old to give up the ghost—and that's a good thing.

If you ever plan to know what life is like on the other side of the sugar addiction that weighs down the version of you that is ready to step up and thrive, you're going to have to listen to that Gut Intelligence at some point. You will have to put aside all the stories that lead to one inevitable conclusion: *I could never do that.* It will mean handing control over to the part of you that is willing to risk discovering that the promise of sugar, all these years, has been a big, fat lie.

I could be way off here—and correct me if I am—but just maybe you've been searching for something this sensible, this simple, and this powerful.

INTERVIEW WITH ALUMNI
Shauna Davis

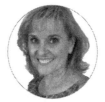

"You'll never know until you try."
—Shauna Davis

Shauna Davis, 50, has been sugar free almost six months at the time of this interview. She is currently a school teacher, positioning herself to go back into dentistry, in which she previously worked as a dental assistant. She has two sons, 25, and 22, as well as three step-children ages, 13, 15, and 17.

What do five kids think about their mom/stepmom being sugar free?
They think it's an oddity, really. My two sons are proud of me. My step-son just shakes his head and narrows his eyes and looks at me. And my step-daughters aren't interested in cutting sugar out of their lives. I don't think it's something that kids really think about. I am doing it because I really want to live a long time. I try to get my husband on board, but he's kind of kicking and screaming.

Why did the 50-year-old mother of five decide that sugar free is a good idea?
I was tired of it controlling me. There were things that people didn't know I was doing. I was keeping it to myself. I would go to the store and buy dessert for everybody and then I got in the car and it called to me. Little Debbie's Cakes or Hostess Ding Dongs and I would think,

"I bought them for the kids... but I like these, too, so I'm just going to eat one." By the time I got into my driveway, maybe only two were left. I'm thinking, "I can't take a box with three Ding Dongs into the house because the kids are going to question me. I'd have to say I ate them and then they'd ask, "How come you only let us eat one at a time and you can eat nine at a time?" Well, because I'm a big fat eater. [Laughs] Then I'm putting myself down but...

I hear you saying that about yourself and I hear you getting sad. You're not alone in that. You know, there are millions of people who do that. I'm two plus years sugar free and I can still find a Reese's peanut butter wrapper—I guarantee you—somewhere in my office, my car, or in my golf bag.

Yes. I'm finding old wrappers in purses and stuff. I was going through some things to go to Goodwill and I found candy wrappers. They were hidden away so that nobody knew I'd eaten them. I simply slid the wrappers down to the bottom of the purse or coat pockets.

How was your sugar intake before you decided to try 30 Days Sugar Free?

Now that I've gotten to be a real good label reader, I realize I was probably ingesting more than I thought. I didn't always have to have something sweet every day. But I probably was getting it because I was eating cereal and it's in every single cereal.

I would have the greatest intentions and then I would arrive at a buffet. Well, that was it. I didn't pick just one thing at a buffet—do I want this one or that one? No. I came back with a plate of a piece of every single one of those things because I was always afraid that I was going to miss out on something. So I wanted to taste everything.

If there was a cake with frosting and big roses? I would joke with my friend about which one of us was going to get the corner piece with two sides of frosting and all the roses! I grew up like that.

How has your sleep been affected by this change in your diet?

I fall asleep when it's bedtime now! I'm tired at the end of a day and I don't have that afternoon slump anymore. I used to drink those little caffeine packets that you put into water. It was an orange drink and each packet had 80 mg of caffeine. I would have one of those in the morning when I first woke up and then about 1 o'clock in the afternoon I'd have another one. So, all that caffeine and aspartame—I was addicted to those big time.

In going 30 Days Sugar Free, was there something that was easier than you thought it would be? Did you have some story in your head that this was going to be impossible?

Honestly, just being able to walk by the dessert tables—now that's easier than I thought it was going to be. I chose December 1st to start! I'm used to eating fudge and making fudge and cookies for everybody. I thought, "If I'm going to do it, this is going to be a good test." Then again, December to me was just like any month. Like I said, if I'm going to go to a party where there's a bunch of desserts, it's going to be like a holiday to me anyway! I was anyone's gal if there was something sugary to eat.

Was there any part of it that has been harder than you thought it would be?

What's harder is that grocery shopping takes longer. If you are going to get packaged things, you are going to have to read the labels. Restaurants are a challenge. Unless you are going to get a steak, or a piece of fish, or a chicken breast or whatever, and season it all yourself. That's what I do. I've always loved fruits and vegetables so having grilled vegetables and fruit as the side is such a treat.

You sound like a very social person. How has the social aspect of being at a party changed?

I actually feel like an evangelist at times! I want to start sharing it with people. I want to tell them, "Don't put that in your mouth," but I don't. If people ask, "Are you going to have any of these desserts?" I say, "No, I don't eat sugar now." They react with, "Oh, really? Not even a little bit?" So I look for something else.

I am in the church choir and a couple was moving and so we put together a little party for them. Some kind soul brought a tray of veggies and dip. I didn't have the dip but I did grab a cup and loaded it with celery and carrots! That was my favorite choice. I had something in my hand. In a party situation it seems you have to hold something in your hand.

Right at that point, does the social interaction change for you? Do you still feel like you have relationships with people at parties? Is there a loss because you are not eating sugar?
I don't feel any loss at all. I still want to go because I like people and I like interacting with them. I just don't eat everything that they are eating. And like I said, I almost feel like I should be saving them from what they are doing but I don't. It has to be an individual decision. It has to come from within.

What surprised you about being sugar free? What changes in your life do you notice that have you asking, "Holy cow... was that tied to all the sugar I was eating?"
My joints don't ache. I can still feel that I have a little bit of swelling, but it doesn't hurt and it's not like it used to be. I mentioned that I don't have an afternoon slump like I used to. I've always been a good water drinker and now I do even more. When I first wake up in the morning I drink 16 ounces and I refill my 20 ounce bottle at work many times every day.

That's so great. Six months in, do you feel like this is a natural lifestyle for you?
I never feel like I have to seek out sugar. If I do want something sweet, I grab some dried mango. I love those. I also keep bananas in the freezer and use them to make ice cream by blending them up with a bit of unsweetened cocoa powder! I don't eat that all the time. A piece of fruit is my go-to. I know when I've had enough for the day. That is very new for me!

I was a formula baby. My mom wasn't able to nurse for whatever reason. The doctors told her that formula is better. So I'm sure I was getting sugar at a very early age through the formula. She was told that to get me to drink water, she should add sugar into the water. I got right on the treadmill.

I've heard you say that getting control over sugar was a big driver in doing this challenge. Was weight loss also a driver for you?

Yes, most definitely because I had been trying to lose weight and I was at a plateau. Whether it's age or post-menopausal, I think my body is just naturally hanging onto stuff. I lost about five pounds in the first five days. Just getting rid of the obvious stuff—protein bars, those drinks. My weight, and everything about me, is much healthier now. And my skin is better. My pores are smaller.

What would you say to someone who says, "That all sounds good but I can't picture myself doing it"?

I'd say, "You never know until you try." I never thought that I was going to be successful. I thought, "I'll do it for 30 days and see what happens." I started on December 1st and Christmas was on my Day 25!

I ate the turkey, the vegetables, and the salad, but I did not miss out on anything. By that time, I was over the addiction to sugar. After the first initial week, then two weeks, and then three weeks, I just felt so good. Ultimate Christmas gift!

You are an incredible inspiration. Any plans to bring sugar back into your life?

No. Once the 30 days were up, I realized there was no reason to go back. It's not worth it. It's not worth it at all. Both of my grandfathers died of heart disease. That plagues me. I needed to do something better. I didn't want that to happen to me. I just don't want that in my future.

I got onto this bandwagon and plan to live in good health for a long time. I want it for everybody. That's what I feel like when I want to tell people in the grocery store, "Get that out of your cart. What are you thinking?"

CHAPTER 2
How We Got Here

Since its humble beginning, sugar has touched our lives and affected our history: global battles, economics, slavery, industrialization, a high-priority of Hitler's regime, an anti-apartheid embargo, and an addiction that is responsible for varying levels of physical and mental suffering for so many human beings.

It was best said by the Beatles in their song, *I Should Have Known Better*, when they screamed, "Give me more, hey hey hey, give me more!" Although the lads were talking about love, the sentiment is equally applicable to sugar.

While the exact date is unknown when a man first walked through an open field, saw what looked like an 8-foot tall sprig of asparagus, and broke it open, it's indisputable that we are still enjoying the rush he experienced with that first lick of the sugarcane.

I laugh thinking about what that first man might have said upon returning to the village. I'm guessing the gist of it was something like this (insert your own dialect and inflection): "Put down the mud, leaves, and bugs mama, you're not going to believe what I just found!"

That moment began a movement in the human race that changed lives. Economy, geography, topography, environment, government, human rights, commerce, longevity, and even hierarchy—every part of the human experience was altered when sugar became part of the equation.

The "fine spice," as it was referred to during the medieval period, has a history that dates back to at least 8,000 BC in New Guinea. A few thousand years later, sugar made its way west to Indonesia, the Philippines, and Northern India.

The History of Sugar

There isn't going to be a quiz, or anything like that, but let me highlight a few of the more important dates and places in sugar's sordid past en route to your 64 oz. soft drink. For a thorough and gripping account of sugar's history, I highly recommend *Sugar: A Bittersweet History*, by Elizabeth Abbott.

500-ish BC – Sugar hit India and the creative manufacturers in that region devised "cooled sugar syrup" which was molded and distributed in the shape of large, flat bowls. This process left sugar in a form that was simple to transport and trade.

300-ish BC – Alexander the Great (yeah, you knew he would have a part in this!) was among the first in Europe to experience the "honey powder" that his troops brought back from India. Perhaps old Alex was more of a savory guy because the entire continent didn't really embrace sugar until after the Crusades, some 1,000 years later.

400-ish AD – Back to the brains of India where the Imperial Guptas found a way to turn sugarcane juice into granulated crystals. EUREKA! Trade of sugar became very popular in this region and these white cakes of "stone honey" were expensive and highly prized.

600-ish AD – "Made in China" was first stamped on a product as they established their sugarcane plantations using technology learned from the kind people of India. That stamp is omnipresent all these centuries later.

800 – 900 AD – An agricultural revolution in Arab countries led to Muslim countries in the Middle East and Asia duplicating the production methods of India.

1,000 — 1,200 AD – Europe re-entered the sugar game and this time it stuck. Their so-called *Golden Age of Discovery* was frosted when the soldiers of the Crusades brought back the "sweet salt."

1,400s – Growing sugarcane required vast amounts of sun and water. The first plantations in Central America were formed.

1,600s – The code on beet sugar was cracked by French agronomist Olivier de Serres. When something is popular, it's always good to find other ways of making it!

1700s – Big turning point here… Get ready. The demand for sugar was flying high and plantations were opened in many areas of Central America and the Caribbean islands. Slaves from Africa were brought to work these plantations under extremely harsh and dangerous conditions.

1800s – Beet sugar factories were built in Germany enabling Europeans to start producing mass amounts of sugar and meet the popular demand. Also in this century, sugar went from being popular to necessary. People were drinking coffee and tea as well as eating jam, candy, chocolate, and other processed foods that required sugar.

1900s – Sugar was an accepted part of the diet to all people around the world. Production became highly industrialized and distribution was cheap and readily available.

1957 – Richard O. Marshall and Earl P. Kooi formulated what is now called high-fructose corn syrup (HFCS) which was cheaper than sugar, wet, readily available, and made from government subsidized corn. This processed form of sugar is now present in countless products today including ketchup, soups, cereals, pasta sauces, and soda.

The use of HFCS has been linked to obesity, learning disability and memory, high blood pressure, and cardiovascular disease, just to name a few of the costs we pay for this sweet concoction.

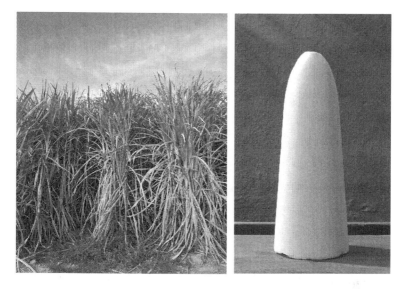

1975 – The book, *Sugar Blues,* by William Dufty, was one of the first of its kind to talk about the history of sugar and the harmful effects of sugar on the human body.

2014 – Movies such as *Fed Up* and others like it reveal research and updated information on the state of our society and its relationship to sugar.

What a journey, right? With the increasing ease to secure and consume sugar, the potential for overdose was predestined. Nothing about sugar consumption is designed for satisfaction nor completion. A binge usually ends when the product is finished, or the user walks away in disgust.

Sugar and Fiber

Originally, to enjoy the sweetness of sugar, one was required to chew on the cane. This action would soften the fiber and, mixed with the saliva in the mouth, release the natural sweetness of the plant. It required a lot of work to get even a small amount of sugar into one's system. In those days, weight gain, or anything even close to obesity, wasn't likely from such a small amount of sugar mixed with the active lifestyle which included hunting, gathering, and working the land.

Industrialization streamlined the process by putting sugar into sugar cones and sugar loafs. Both of these forms required consumers to use a tool, called sugar nips, to break off pieces. These tools were quite elaborate—pliers mounted in a box with holes on the bottom where the sugar could fall onto a plate or baking dish.

Now there is no such Olympic event required to get a fix of sugar. Pour a bowl of cereal, tear open a granola bar, make a peanut butter and jelly sandwich—even open a jar of "healthy" pasta sauce—and your sugar is served right up. Yogurt, sliced meats, bread, applesauce, shredded cheese, table salt, and just about every beverage imaginable are on the list of foods that get the average person in a first-world country to digest a whopping 130 lbs of sugar each year. I'm not great at the metric system, but that has to be close to 200 kilometers!

The Myths About Fat

In the '70s, the medical establishment believed it had discovered a link between our diets and the rise in weight gain, obesity, and heart disease. Fats in foods were considered the culprit. Medical organizations lobbied the government and new mandates were put in place to cut the amount of fat that was added to everything from hamburgers to crackers.

"They figured it was the fat in foods", says Robert Lustig, an American pediatric endocrinologist at the University of California, San Francisco. Food manufacturers obeyed and, as Lustig says, "When you take the fat out of food, it tastes like cardboard. What did they do? They added high-fructose corn syrup and sucrose."

While advances in medical technology were keeping us alive longer, the amount of sugar and processed food we were eating was killing us faster. Sugar fattened us up—pills, diets, and snake oils were invented to keep us thin. When sugar took its toll on the skin and teeth, surgeries were created to tighten the wrinkles and replace the enamel.

As it turns out, "fat" was a bit too broad a stroke with the sword. Some fats are necessary for healthy living.

"Functional practitioners that focus on the true underlying causes of dysfunction in the body have known all along that fats are not the culprits that create chronic illness and inflammation," says Victoria LaFont, Nutritional Therapy Practitioner. "I'm glad to see that healthy fats such as butter and coconut oil are finally getting the positive media attention they deserve. It's a biochemical fact that appropriate lipids and amino acids actually build immunity, create sound cellular structure, and hormonally satiate us so that we don't crave the foods of commerce—namely, processed sugars. Want to give up sugar? Eat butter."

Depression to Entitlement

The amount of sugar we eat is taking a prominent place in global conversations about health—and not a moment too soon. The U.N. Secretary General declared that non-communicable diseases, such as diabetes, heart disease, obesity, cancer, and Alzheimer's, are a bigger threat to the entire world, developed and developing, than is infectious disease.

In the 2014 documentary film *Fed Up*, narrator Katie Couric states that by 2034, 95% of the American population will be overweight or obese. (Remember the floating blobs of humans in another popular movie, *Wally*?) And just in case you're not connecting the dots, obesity and being overweight are both non-communicable diseases.

Our addiction to sugar is ancient. You did nothing but show up at a time in history when a flag with the word "More" was waving wildy in the wind. It's not your fault that you are popping a donut into your mouth at 7AM, or drinking a soda the size of your head with lunch, or eating four servings (one pint) of Ben & Jerry's at 11PM.

During the Great Depression, families learned to ration, scrimp, and even go without much of what was considered normal. Culturally, we struggle with the juxtaposition of, "This could happen again," and, "We were deprived for long enough—eat all you want." While the previous generation of depression survivors saw the value of moderation, baby boomers feel entitled to the entire buffet of options— money, possessions, love, and yes, sugar.

Our sweet tooth snuck up on us and was granted looser reins in perfect harmony with greater supply, cheaper alternatives, and sloppy research. Answering the call for more sugar, big food's commitment to making it cheap and available has brought us to the threshold of a monumental decision: what role do we, going forward, want sugar to play in our lives and the lives our children?

Parting Shot from 13th Century Poet and Mystic Rumi:

Don't Go Back to Sleep
The breeze at dawn has secrets to tell you.
Don't go back to sleep.
You must ask for what you really want.
Don't go back to sleep.
People are going back and forth across the door sill
where the two worlds touch.
The door is round and open.
Don't go back to sleep.

Arlene Krantz

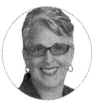

"I realized that if I make up my mind I'll do it. If you make up your mind, it will happen. There will be ups and downs. But nothing will stop you." —Arlene Krantz

Arlene Krantz is a vivacious 74-year old grandmother who lives in West Hollywood, California. She has two daughters and is a very happy grandmother of seven grandkids. She loves to hang out with friends and have dinner but doesn't like small talk. She has been vegan and sugar free for three months at the time of this interview.

What substitutions have you made in your diet since going sugar free?

I love to drink wine, but I would wake up the next day with a sugar hangover. I grew up in Philadelphia and also love ice cream. But then I went vegan and wouldn't eat the dairy. So I found a coconut milk ice cream and had it every night. I became addicted. Then I'd wake up the next day feeling groggy. I said, "I can't do that anymore."

Once I made up my mind to be sugar free, after meeting Barry... I said, "I've got to do this." What I do now is take a frozen banana, unsweetened cocoa powder, and chopped almonds and put it in my little mixer. That's my ice cream.

Normally, I drink tea with honey. Well, honey is sugar. I decided to try it without honey. And it wasn't so bad. I love tea, so why not? Then one day I decided to try honey in it again. I could feel and taste that honey in my body.

Wow!
It tasted good but my body was asking, "What are you doing to me?" Once I made up my mind, I just went 100%.

When I want something sweet, my neighbor has a fig tree. All that natural sugar. So good.

Do you feel any difference when you eat fruit with a natural sugar versus something like the brownies with added processed sugar?
I can't even think about the brownies because I know it will just destroy my body. Figs don't have the same effect.

I heard you say giving up honey in tea was easier than you thought it would be. What else did you give up?
I gave up chai lattes... I did try them sugar free but it's still sweet. Not always sure what's in it.

There's a really great automatic translation you can do in your head when you hear sugar free. My brain hears it as a "probable chemical storm."
I stopped sodas ages ago. One time, though, I had pizza and I said, "Okay, I'm going to have a Diet Coke." Now I don't drink Diet Coke. When I got it, I looked at the glass and said, "I can't do this." I poured it down the sink. I'm going to take this chemical that burns holes and corrodes metal and put it in my body? Are you crazy, Arlene?

It's good for cleaning pennies and toilets though. I don't say throw it away, I just say repurpose it. So what makes this challenge worth the effort for someone your age?
I have seven grandkids so I'm up there. But the thing is, I need to keep my body in good shape. It's very easy these days to be diabetic and I don't want that. Before I went sugar free, I had a blood test and I was borderline diabetic.

Too many people I see are diabetic. My sister is diabetic. It's like an epidemic.

So you are using the good feelings along with a fear tactic to keep you away from sugar. Are you finding adaptations and living mostly a sugar free life?

I started 100%, but sometimes I waver. I was just at the airport after four days of being in a workshop all day long, so I treated myself. I got a coconut milk chocolate Fudgesicle. You know something? It was good but it wasn't as satisfying as it used to be.

Because you knew you were having sugar?

Oh yeah. And it's a huge change to be able to do that on a conscious level.

How do you handle celebrations or parties?

Sometimes I'll eat ahead of time. I'll always ask if there is sugar in something. I made the mistake recently of ordering teriyaki at a Chinese restaurant because they didn't have a lot of vegan choices. The sauce was loaded with sugar, sugar, sugar.

Is there something you learned about yourself from radically reducing the amount of sugar you have in your life?

Well, what I realized about me is that if I make up my mind I'll do it. And that's what people have to really learn is that you just have to make up your mind. If you make up your mind, it will happen. Nothing will stop you. There will be ups and downs.

What I would always tell somebody is, "It's got to be in your head."

Is there anything that surprised you as you were doing it?

What I noticed is how much sugar is out there. I became very conscious of everything that has sugar in it. And I became conscious of the people around me and how we eat so much sugar. It's even in tobacco. No wonder people that are smoking can't give it up. It's got sugar.

You are among the rarities in the world who have chosen a relationship with sugar that is controlled.

There are other ways to satisfy that sweet taste. I make chia pudding with almond milk that has no sugar in it. I grate oranges in it and some vanilla. I always keep bananas in the freezer for dessert as well.

What would you tell someone who's lived their whole life eating sugar and is maybe thinking about doing this?

We all have to go sometime. Now, how do you want to go? Do you want to go with popping pills, having insulin? Do you want to be healthy for the rest of your life? One main benefit is that I feel good about myself. I keep myself healthy. I'm not young, you know.

I want to be different. I want to be an inspiration for everybody around me not to have sugar. What do we need it for? Where? Where do we need it? We don't.

CHAPTER 3
Living in the Habit of Sugar

Are you somewhere that you can see people? Perhaps you're on a train, in a building with a window, or even in a car listening to this book being read aloud. In a moment, I'm going to ask you to stop reading (or listening) and take a look at a random person that you don't know. We are going to play a little game.

The Game of Projection

In this context, projection means the attribution of one's own ideas, feelings, or attitudes to other people. It's part of our operating system as human beings. We see someone and instantly form a story. The brain works very quickly and for this exercise I'm going to ask you to slow it down a bit. We are going look at the act of projection consciously.

Can you imagine what it might be like to be this person you are looking at? Give yourself full permission to dig in and give voice to your reaction (whether silent or spoken). Deeply own every single thought, judgment, feeling, and belief you have about that person you are looking at. Hold nothing back—even if it isn't something you would "normally" think, feel, or say. Keep going until you get to the point where you can feel empathy for this person. Give this at least a minute, hopefully longer. OK... release it all. Poof!

Round One:
Does the person look any different to you right now?

Do you feel differently toward that person?

Is that person any different right now?

Has their life been affected or changed by the exercise you just completed?

Round Two:

Do you look any different after playing Projection?

Do you feel any different?

Are you any different right now?

Has your life been affected by the exercise you just completed?

Alright, why did I just ask you to do that? Because nothing has really changed.

Oh, sure, we can talk about how everything is energy and what you just did altered the course of both your lives. I know that conversation, and it makes for an interesting discussion. Right now, though, I'm talking about actual changes that a video camera would pick up—indisputable actions viewable by an impartial witness. Has anything changed?

That person is still doing the same thing she or he was doing before becoming the object of your exercise. You are still reading or listening to this book. It was a moment in time that left no tangible mark on the world—just like a hundred other thoughts, judgments, and beliefs you have every single day of your life.

We'd spend less time worrying about what others think about us if we realized how seldom they do.

Yet we often let the thoughts, judgments, and beliefs of others influence our behavior. How can this be? You just spent a minute or so judging the heck out of someone and they didn't even know it happened. The guy was standing there looking into a shop window and you developed a whole story about his diet, the stain on his shirt, his girlfriend (who wasn't even there!), his financial story, what he was thinking about—and he didn't even know you existed.

Poof!

For you to walk any path that looks different is, to varying degrees, a threat to those who know you. Your desire to change or recreate yourself is a bright and shiny mirror to those in your life who want to make a change. Many times they will find it easier to help you temper your lofty goals than it is for them to rise up and draw a line in the sand. Imagine that—your desire for self-improvement is an affront to many friends and family who love you dearly.

It Happens Everywhere

This was posted from Mary in an online group for 30 Days Sugar Free:

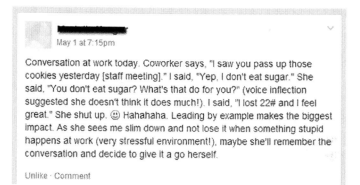

The person who shot off this comment didn't spend a lot of time thinking about our Mary. Instead, it instantly became an opportunity to convince herself that going sugar free wasn't worth the effort. That's much easier than facing the daunting and devastating truth that she could probably benefit in many areas of her life if she tried a sugar free challenge.

The fact that she noticed Mary passing up the cookies—and that it stayed with her overnight—is a powerful indicator that her expectations weren't met and this rocked her a bit. Her expectations were that when a plate of cookies arrived, everyone should eat them. Mary passing on the cookies brought up an emotion for her co-worker. My experience as a coach leads me to believe that it was actually three emotions: fear (is there something wrong with me for taking one when Mary isn't?), anger (why isn't Mary taking a cookie!?), and ultimately, sadness (why am I taking a cookie when I'm not hungry?).

Of course, we are creatures of habit. Habits allow us to stay alive and get things done. They are also why many people die too soon and don't get anything done! We have this remarkable—albeit treacherously challenging—ability to change our habits. While the logical parts of our brain might be very clear that we'd like to change a certain behavior, there is the habitual cycle that fights tooth-and-nail to keep doing the same things in the same way. If only changing a habit were as simple as wishing it so!

Breaking Down the Habits

Habits come in two main flavors: unconscious and conscious. They show up for different reasons and serve different purposes.

Unconscious Habits – These are the ones that most often come from a place of fear, protection, modeling, or convenience. Often we pick them up when we are small and never bother to send out the eviction notice. They might very well have kept us safe when we were young, but at this point they are just hanging around, keeping us small, and generally wasting our time and energy.

Conscious Habits – These are the domain of achievers. These habits are planned, coordinated, and executed by design. They are usually preceded by some research and education and have to be practiced over some period of time until they become automatic. These are the gold bars of change and achievement. Once a conscious habit is engaged, you are playing your top game and have the capacity to look for another area of your life where you can create the next one.

There is a science behind the study of habits. In his book, *The Power of Habit*, Charles Duhigg shares a framework for understanding how habits work and a guide to experimenting with how they might change. It's very left brain (analytical) and well-written. The three-word abstract of his manuscript is this: cue, habit, reward.

Breaking this cycle for a day is a lesson in patience. It's a seemingly never-ending sequence of catching yourself, changing the behavior, and repeating. You can certainly break a habit for a day, or even several days, but often with a defeated attitude as the old habit still looms. The compounding interest begins paying off after a few days of do-or-die determination. I have designed the 30 day challenge because that amount of time is ample to lick this habit. Based on my own experience and the witnessing and study of thousands of others, I've seen the patterns that are prevalent in those doing the 30 Days Sugar Free challenge.

I've read of 7 and 10 day sugar free challenges. To me, that is when the transformation just starts to get interesting! After 10 days, the body is giving up the ghost, feeling the benefits, and looking at what it can have, instead of what it can't have. That might be the worst time ever to return the body to sugar and let it know that you were just joking—sorry about that! Yikes—no thank you.

Your Amazing Brain

Your brain is a phenomenal machine. It is an expert at protecting you from risking pain and suffering. It is constantly measuring pain and pleasure. Its goal is to keep away the former, and deliver more of the latter. Knowing this makes it very clear why someone who is overweight still wakes up in the morning and eats a chocolate croissant. His brain sees eating it as pleasure and not eating it as pain. Later that morning, however, when the pastry isn't staring him in the face, his brain can recognize the pain and has no visual or other sensory connection to the sweet treat. That is when he thinks, "I shouldn't have eaten that first thing in the morning because it's fattening, bad for my skin, and it makes me crave more sugar."

These are the moments of clarity where someone will swear to never do that again, join a gym, or even throw away whatever is left of the sweet food that gave them the sickening feeling. Any of these three options are good for the analytical part of the brain. "Hey—good for you! Look at you really taking care of yourself. It's going to be all different from here on out!"

That moment of clarity, however, doesn't stand a chance once the sugar crash ends and you are standing around hungry. Gyms are profitable because of this cycle and the fact that 67% of the people with memberships never use the gym! By the time you change clothes to work out and drive to the gym, the brain has already set its sights on the candy bar that requires no special preparation. Chances are you'll cave because the brain seeks to gain pleasure even more than it does to avoid pain.

It's possible that for you, a lot of this might not apply. In your hands is a book that most people will never hold. They saw the title and made some sound that surely sprayed spittle out onto the other books on the shelf, or even onto their own computer screen. I don't know what got you here. Perhaps it had something to do with physical, mental, or emotional pain stemming from your habits around sugar. That's a powerful motivator if the personal costs are high enough to carry you through.

I can hear you asking, "Why does all of this matter in a discussion about living in the habit of sugar?" Simple answer, and here it is: there are only two people who can get in your way as you attempt to redefine your relationship to sugar. Anyone who tosses a well-timed judgment, feeling, or belief your way. And yourself.

In the first half of this chapter we addressed the influence of others. Now, let's turn to the bigger, more powerful person. You.

Your Role in Changing Habits

There is a phrase that gets tossed around a lot in the conversation of 30 Days Sugar Free: *I could never do that.* Many times it's instantaneous—without even a second to contemplate if it's true or not. Maybe you said it when you saw the name of this book!

Let's look at that definitive statement and see if there is some wiggle room that could lead to the possibility of not only a 30 Day Sugar Free challenge, but even bigger and more important challenges that you'll surely encounter in your life.

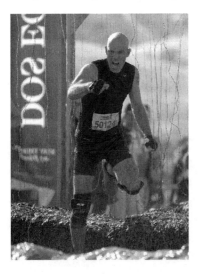

The Risk of "I Could Never Do That"

This picture was taken on September 29, 2012. That was seven months to the day after I said, "I could never do that," about quitting sugar, and four months to the day after I said, "I could never do that," in response to an invitation to join a team of friends doing a Tough Mudder race in Lake Tahoe, CA. The picture caught me running through the final challenge in the 10-mile race that included 26 British Military obstacles. Those wires are laced with 10,000 volts and at the instant this picture was snapped, I was feeling the love from one of them.

I could never do that.

When was the last time you said those five words? Maybe it was watching one of those dramatic talent shows on television, or seeing people dive off boulders in Acapulco, or watching a quadriplegic navigate through a mall by blowing into a straw on her wheelchair.

I could never do that.

There are at least three unintended consequences that happen when that sentence falls from my lips—and each of them have a big effect on how I show up in the world:

I cheat myself out of fully imagining what the experience not only feels like but what it could mean to me long-term. Every adventure in my life has opened the door for more that is new, challenging, and makes me a bigger version of myself.

I send a very clear message to myself that new experiences are too scary, not worth consideration, and it's best to just keep looking forward.

I condition myself to play smaller in the world. The mental shutdown that comes from the utterance of those words is a strong vote for me staying stuck in the same places, lazy in the same ways, and limited by the same beliefs.

Does any of that ring true for you, too?

I could never do that.

That phrase is a reinforcement that beats the life out of my inner adventurer. It's one word away from "I could do that," which sends a completely different message to every cell of my being.

So, next time you see or hear something that sounds extraordinary, difficult, challenging, scary, or down-right stupid (I'm thinking Tough Mudder with that last one), take a moment and contemplate what gifts the experience could offer, how it could empower you to do something even bigger, or how it could change the world.

From this chapter, I want you to take away that there are two big tripping points you will encounter in changing any habit in your life: yourself, and anyone else. The first you have ultimate control over through the stories you tell yourself and the beliefs you hold as true.

The second can only offer advice and guidance that has been distorted by the prism of their own experience.

What you see, hear, and read has great power. Your thoughts influence your feelings which affect your actions and determine your results. In all areas of your life, better input leads to better output.

The 30 Days Sugar Free challenge launches a pinball into well-choreographed habits—yours and those people in your life. Expect the dance of confusion, bliss, resentment, and renewal. Those emotions are the blankets that shield you from change, and also pad the unavoidable bumps en route to transformation.

Andrew Smith

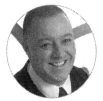

"This has turned from a project into a lifestyle.
I am Mr. Joe Public. If I can do it, anyone can do it."
—*Andrew Smith*

A ndrew Smith lives in Hong Kong and is 53 years old. He has been married since 1990 and has four children between the ages of 12 and 24. He has a most interesting career—he creates world class balloon sculptures and performs around the world. Of course, this creates a special challenge of living sugar free on the road. In this interview Andrew shares his story and what keeps him going.

When did you start 30 Days Sugar Free?
January 1, 2014. Right into the new year!

What was the thought process that led you to do this?
I knew I was eating too much sugar and I knew I really needed to lose weight. So the two things came together and I decided to knock out the sugar—100% no sugar. Starting January 1st, I already had Christmas out of the way and I thought I could focus on the weight loss and going sugar free at the same time.

What was your sugar life like before you started this?
Up until the middle of last summer, I was drinking about four or five

pints of tea a day, and I'd have three or four sugars in each mug. I gradually tried to ease off the tea and knock out the sugar, but I was still eating bags of candy. When I was traveling, I had to have a bag next to me. I was planning to just have one or two pieces, and then I'd get to my destination and there would be nothing left.

I'd go to Starbucks for a coffee and I'd order an extra large hot chocolate. I'd have one of those a day. And, of course, chocolate in the evening. I was probably the biggest one in the house for saying, "Should we get some chocolate?" I didn't drink too many canned or soda drinks, but it was more the chocolate side of things.

It sounds like it was a slow drip throughout your entire waking period.
It was. I had a big ah-ha moment when I was traveling on an overseas trip. I carried a 10 kilo bag of candy in my hand all day. Two or three airports, walking around with a 10 kilo bag, and I thought, "This is heavy! This is really, really heavy!" I realized that was exactly how much weight I was carrying around on my stomach!

There was also strain on my knee—an old knee injury—and I was again, "Ten kilos? That is phenomenal." I've got to lose that.

That's what got me thinking, "I've got to do something about it." I saw the 30 Days Sugar Free challenge and I jumped in.

Brilliant. A really smart way to do it.
It seemed to work well for me. I knew I needed to reduce it before quitting it for 30 days. I started cutting it out, which is quite tough over Christmas with my family, with loads of chocolate and everything else around. It was tough, but I managed to work my way to making January 1st the easiest day.

What did friends and family say when you were going through this?
My kids were overjoyed because they said, "Great, there's more for us." My wife was very supportive. She said, "Yup, I'll do the same." And she has reduced her sugar intake greatly. She hasn't stopped altogether. There is still a lot of chocolate in the house, but I don't touch it. The children help, too. If they see something that may contain sugar, they

will eat it and say, "Dad, it's got sugar in it. Don't eat it!" They try to help me and remind me. They've been very supportive.

My friends have noticed I've lost weight. One of them asked me not to tell his wife that I'm on a sugar free diet. He doesn't want to be forced to go on it himself.

There's a mindset in this and I know you talk about it. It's not *what you can't have* so much as *what you choose to have*. This is my life. This is how I feel better when I don't eat it and this is how I eat now.

My struggle was always the coffee shop, the bun, the cake, and the hot chocolate. By changing the places I visit, I don't have that tendency to go and grab a sticky bun or something.

And the other thing I do at Starbucks is that I go straight up to the register, grab an apple and a bottle of water. No more waiting in the long lines!

That's part of the mindset. It's changing the environment that I'm in but also focusing on, as you say, what you can buy and what you can make.

Do you feel like you've lost anything?

Well, I've lost that 10 kilos!

I also ruined a kitchen table by drilling holes through it when making extra notches in my belt!

As far as food-wise, I don't really think I've lost out. I'm not missing the chocolates. My health is greatly improved and my well-being throughout the day is improved because I've had no sugar for breakfast. I don't have the highs and lows that the sugar created previously. I don't go into shakes at 11 o'clock in the morning. I don't suffer from withdrawals throughout the day. I don't feel hungry all the time. So I don't think I've lost anything. I certainly gained a far more stable blood sugar level.

Is there anything that you haven't mentioned that surprised you, that you learned about yourself, or that you've been able to do in your life since you've been clean of sugar?

I've been surprised that I managed to keep it going beyond 30 days. This has turned from a project into a lifestyle. It has also helped with knowing that I can achieve other things as well. This has been part of a process of keeping my mind clear and focusing on what I want to achieve in other areas of my life, with other objectives.

It's proved to me that if I could give up sugar, which I thought was quite tough at the beginning, I could do other things just as easily by focusing on them. I've managed to achieve so much more work this year because I've focused on it and looked at the positive side of things rather than—I need the sugar fix.

The hardest part of all of this, I would say, has been reading the labels on the stuff I buy in the shop because it's in such small print. I've had to walk around now with a magnifying glass just because I can't see it. Or I keep passing it over to my children to read.

I would say I'm 99% sugar free. I might get some in the odd slice of bread, or a small bit in a sauce that's added to something I've ordered in the restaurant.

Let's just be clear for the sake of people reading this. You told us you were traveling through airports with a bag of sugar next to your side and it was gone when you arrived. I've seen those Starbucks drinks. So now you occasionally think, "I'm going to eat a piece of bread!" Is that right? You are the 1%, my friend!
Well, if you look at it like that, it's been pretty amazing.

Did you buy new pants? Ten kilos! That's a lot of weight.
It is. I'm having to put belts on and I can actually take my trousers off at the end of the day by undoing the belt and just letting the unbuckled trousers fall to the floor. My target is to get down to another 10 kilos, so I'm trying not to buy too many clothes now.

How has your life changed in terms of physical exercise?
Walking or swimming has been my exercise. Although I have to tell you, last weekend I ran a 10k!

I am still eating other foods so I have to burn the calories off. And I quite like walking. It's a great time to think and focus on work and projects.

I've cut down all the things that I felt I needed to have to keep me going and I'm a buzzing man. I'm buzzing.

Would you say you're an exceptional person, or could somebody reading this say, "That could be me?"

[Laughs]. No way. I've got the name "Andrew Smith"—the surname is very common, very average, and I've always been Mr. Average throughout my life. There's nothing different about me. I am Mr. Joe Public. If I can do it, anyone can do it. There's nothing special about me apart from the fact that I decided to have a go at it and stuck with it. I'm normal. I'm a normal fellow.

You're a huge success story in this. I'm so happy for you.

Oh, thank you for introducing me to 30 Days Sugar Free, Barry. I really appreciate it.

CHAPTER 4
Food 101

I'm not a doctor or a nutritionist. I don't want to mislead you with regard to my qualifications in broaching a chapter called Food 101.

Like you, I have danced with food my entire life. Perhaps unlike you, I have spent the last few years seriously considering what I eat, studying experts, interviewing authorities, and noting the effect that different foods have on my physical, emotional, and mental health.

In this chapter, I share the most basic explanation of how our diet defines who we are. This is not a book about nutrition. I offer this chapter to help you understand that processed and refined sugar isn't a necessary part of your diet. If you are looking for a brilliant book about nutrition and diet, I recommend *The China Study: The Most Comprehensive Study of Nutrition Ever Conducted and the Startling Implications for Diet, Weight Loss, and Long-term Health* by Thomas Campbell.

The Potato Talk

It's funny, but one of the first questions people ask when I talk about this challenge concerns carbohydrates that turn into sugar in the body. Would those be allowed on the challenge? I was eating so many Snickers and Kit Kat bars that my focus was squarely on the refined and processed sugar. I couldn't imagine that people could be so clean as to worry if a potato might be a violation. Through my lens, there were bigger fish to fry!

However, let's dig into the carbohydrate story and get clear on how it relates to nutrition.

There are three types of carbohydrates: simple sugar, starch, and fiber. Fiber passes through the digestive track because we don't have the enzymes necessary to digest and convert it to sugar. Think of fiber as a security officer whose job is to make sure everything keeps progressing towards the exit door. Graphic, I know, and very important, indeed!

The first two types of carbohydrates, simple sugars and starch, are broken down into sugars that the body uses for energy.

Simple Sugars

Some foods contain simple sugars which don't need to be further broken down during digestion. The three main simple sugars are glucose, fructose, and galactose. Glucose is found in honey and fruit. Fructose is found in fruits, vegetables, and honey. Galactose is found in plants. Glucose and galactose are easily absorbed, but some people have difficuly absorbing fructose if it isn't accompanied by glucose or galactose.

Compound Sugars

Compound Sugars include sucrose, a combination of fructose and glucose; lactose, a combination of galactose and glucose; and maltose, which is a combination of two glucose molecules. Sucrose is found in sugar and maple syrup, lactose is found in milk and maltose is found in—wait for it—malt, fruits and grains. During digestion, the enzymes break the bonds between the sugar molecules to turn compound sugars into simple sugars.

Starches

Plants form starches, which are also called complex carbohydrates, by stringing together sugars. When you eat starchy foods, the starches are broken down into sugars—including glucose, maltotriose, and maltose—by an enzyme called amylase. This enzyme is found in your saliva and small intestine. Other enzymes further break down these compound sugars into simple sugars such as maltase, lactase, sucrase, and isomaltase.

High Fructose Corn Syrup (HFCS)

In my exhaustive research of High Fructose Corn Syrup (HFCS), I discovered that it is being added to more and more foods and drinks. There is a big political story behind corn that I'm not going to get into right now. Some of the words that would have starring roles in a full discussion would include: corn, government, lobbyists, subsidies, farmers, fuel source, cheaper than sugar, and plenty of land to grow it. Suffice it to say that the major players make for interesting and unlikely bedfellows.

I did find one website that couldn't say enough good things about high fructose corn syrup—and it's their job. The Corn Refiners Association loves the stuff.

On the site is a short video and the message boils down to three main benefits: HFCS is cheap, convenient, and wet. Is it wrong to expect more from what we put in our bodies?

You can see the video by going to the online member area. http://ILoveMeMoreThanSugar.com

I assure you one thing about HFCS—nothing will go wrong with your body or health by simply eliminating it from your diet. Check the labels and just say no thank you. You know what else is cheap, convenient, and wet that your body actually needs? Water!

Why Water?

During a 30 Days Sugar Free challenge, I ask people to drink a lot of water. So much of the time we can squelch the calling for something sweet by enjoying two glasses of water. During the early days of the challenge your body is detoxifying from sugar, and water is the most efficient way of moving the toxins through. To make clear to you visual learners, water should be going in and coming out every 15 minutes during your 30 Days Sugar Free challenge.

You lose a lot of water just by being alive! Sweat, elimination, and evaporation (as you breathe and through your skin) can leave you dehydrated and that is the runway for poor decisions, short tempers, foggy thinking, and so many other undesirable conditions. Dehydration also clears a path for sugar cravings because it depletes the body of various minerals and nutrients. Your body is composed of approximately 60% water. If you don't believe me, try making jerky

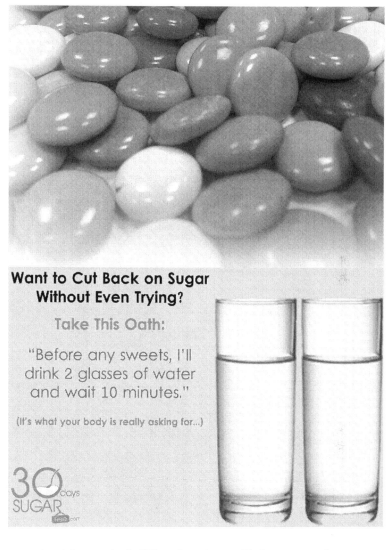

**Want to Cut Back on Sugar
Without Even Trying?**

Take This Oath:

"Before any sweets, I'll
drink 2 glasses of water
and wait 10 minutes."

(It's what your body is really asking for...)

30 days
SUGAR free.com

sometime! One and a half lbs of tri-tip quickly becomes a few ounces
of jerky once you remove the water. I'm not saying you are jerky, but
there are similarities!

Drinking plenty of water will spare you all sorts of unpleasant
reactions including those mentioned above. Your muscles also need
water. Cells that don't maintain a fluid balance shrivel and this can
easily lead to muscle fatigue or cramping.

There are dozens of ways to alter the appearance of the skin including vitamins, make-up, or surgery. A simple and inexpensive answer is water. Dehydration makes your skin look dry and wrinkled. This condition will improve with regular hydration. It's not as sexy nor does it make nearly as exciting a story as a full-blown face lift.

Water is magical for all your organs—from the skin to the kidneys, to the bowels and beyond. Can you agree to the oath shown in the picture? I had that graphic made after the strategy worked so well for me—I hope it works for you, too!

Shooting Down the Additives

This 30 Days Sugar Free challenge is about eliminating the processed and refined sugars from your diet. I don't advocate cutting natural forms of sugar without consulting a health professional. Here we grab our courage and kick the legs out from under the easy targets. Sugar that is added to many foods is addictive, unnecessary, and a luxury that few can afford while hoping to live in a state of excellent health.

Fact is, we have not evolved to the point where we can eat today's high sugar diet and thrive.

So enjoy your fruit, potatoes, a bit of good wine. The changes we are making are big enough. If you want to go deeper into the practice of removing sugars from your diet, wait until the 30 days are finished and then make a new goal.

Calories, Insulin, Fiber, Oh My!

Calories are all alike, whether they come from beef or bourbon, from sugar or starch, or from cheese and crackers. Too many calories are just too many calories.
—Fred Stare, founder and former chair of the Harvard University Nutrition Department

But is that quote true? Maybe Fred Stare, like many Americans, is misinformed.

Calories In/Calories Out

There are diets galore that have you counting calories. The idea is that if you eat less and exercise more, weight loss will ensue. But what most people don't know—including Fred Stare of Harvard—is that this depends on the source of the calories.

When Dr. Richard Lustig, who teaches pediatrics in the Division of Endocrinology at UCSF, was asked, "Is a calorie a calorie?" his answer was, "Not even close." Calories are not interchangeable and the idea that they are has led to a lot of misinformation. It's important to consider the metabolic effects of the calories as well.

There's a lot to learn from Lustig. I have studied many of his interviews and writings and I believe his research will play a big role in the reversal of our sugar pandemic. Below are summaries of his findings that pertain to sugar and the human body.

Fiber

Let's look at 160 calories of almonds and 160 calories of soda. There are two kinds of fiber in almonds—soluble and insoluble.

When you consume food that has both fibers, the insoluble fiber forms a gel on the inside of the intestine—kind of like a bathtub's plastic drain catcher. The soluble fiber is like the hair that gets caught. This barrier of gel reduces the rate of absorption of calories and other nutrients, which move down into the system before being absorbed.

The rise rate of blood glucose is slower and longer, therefore the insulin response is less, and more of what you eat gets delivered to the bacteria in your intestine. We'll find out why that's good in a moment.

No Fiber

How about those 160 calories of soda which are filled with high fructose corn syrup (HFCS)? In HFCS, glucose and fructose are disassociated, so there is no fiber to slow them down. They get absorbed early on in the intestine and go straight to the liver. Your liver gets overwhelmed and that leads to a higher chance of chronic metabolic disease. Plus, the good bacteria are starving.

Big Bags of Bacteria

Lustig calls us "big bags of bacteria with legs." We are each made up of 10 trillion cells. There are 100 trillion bacteria in our intestine. These are huge numbers that I'm not even sure I can visualize. And these bacteria have to eat something. They eat what you eat.

Some bacteria make bad things like endotoxins, which happens when the gut can't do the job it's supposed to do. When the endotoxins get absorbed, inflammation occurs. This is what drives chronic metabolic diseases. Feed the good bacteria—you don't get endotoxins.

What can change bad to good is fiber.

So Where's the Fiber?

Many people think cereal is a good source of fiber. Cereal is filled with sugar. The box may say, "Low fat, high fiber." That's a lie. They may say "Made with whole grains." Another lie. The product may have started with a whole grain but it got pulverized in the process. The FDA has no definition of whole grain. The cereal manufacturer also most likely used refined corn flour which is high on the glycemic index and isn't a very healthy grain.

Here are some good sources of fiber:
- Nuts – almonds, pecans, and walnuts have the most.
- Brown rice – skip the white – all the fiber's gone.
- Whole grains – whole-wheat bread, pasta, etc.
- Vegetables – the crunchier, the better.
- Beans – burritos, chili, soup, salads, etc.
- Popcorn – a fun source of fiber and excellent transporter of flavors.
- Baked potato with skin – the fiber is in the skin.
- Berries – all those seeds, plus the skin, give great fiber to any berry. Try freezing raspberries on a hot day.
- Oatmeal – Steel cut or regular, both have good fiber.

The Quality of Calories

Inside the pancreas, beta cells make the hormone called insulin.

Our metabolism does not decide to burn or store body fat based on calories. It makes these decisions based on the hormones those calories trigger. That is why the quality of calories matters so much. Higher-quality calories trigger body fat-*burning* hormones while low-quality calories trigger body fat-*storing* hormones.

What are Good Fats and Why Eat Them?

In the chapter, *How We Got Here,* I quoted Nutritional Therapy Practitioner Victoria LaFont about the importance of good fats. "Fat releases hormones to the brain that tell us we are satiated and full. Fatty acid deficiency is the number one deficiency in the United States. We need more good fats."

Good fats. Let that combination of words find a resting place in your brain because there has been so much tied to fats being bad. Good fats are the naturally occurring, traditional fats that haven't been damaged by high heat, refining, processing or other man-made tampering, such as "partial hydrogenation." The best of these kinds of fats are found in fish, nuts, avocados, seeds, and even fresh creamery butter.

Here is Victoria's list of Must Have Fats:
- For cooking – coconut oil and pasteurized butter
- For salad dressings – olive oil (do not cook olive oil on high heat)
- For supplementing a healthy diet – a high quality fish oil and pumpkin seed oil (refrigerated in dark bottles, eaten within six months of production)
- Avocado – yes, it's the poster child for good fat and for a good reason. It's the perfect snack, right from its very own package.

Protein

With any discussion of sugar, it's important to touch on protein as well. Protein builds, maintains, and replaces the tissues in your body. Muscles, organs, and the immune system are all made up, for the most part, of protein. Our bodies convert the protein we eat into specialized protein molecules that have very specific jobs.

Starting your day with protein is a huge gift you can give yourself. Protein is a building block of cells in our body that rebuild muscles, strengthen bones, and support healthy blood and organs. Morning protein also sets a very low expectation for sugar throughout the day and will keep us feeling full for a longer period of time.

Leptin and Insulin

We have an obesity epidemic in America. Is this just because our collective will has gone soft? If we get a good motivational coach, won't we get off the couch and exercise? Not really. Let's talk about a hormone called Leptin. It's nicknamed the "satiety hormone" and acts as an appetite thermometer, telling the brain, "You've had enough to eat."

But high quantities of sugar intake can throw this off, causing *Leptin resistance*. This means the cells in the brain no longer read the Leptin signals and instead believe that the body is starving—no matter how much food the person eats. The brain then goes on high alert to increase energy storage, instigating powerful cravings for high-fat, high-sugar foods because they produce immediate energy. It also sends the message to conserve energy.

You can see it—that classic picture of the overweight person on the couch flipping channels and eating Oreos, powerless to make a change.

To top it off—there's the insulin issue. Those high sugar diets lead to repeated spikes in insulin. Not only does a high amount of insulin try to change energy to fat, it can also lead to *insulin resistance*. This is when the cells have been so bombarded by insulin they no longer respond to it. Insulin is the blocker of Leptin signaling. Too much insulin triggers Leptin resistance! Can you see a vicious cycle?

And what makes insulin levels go up? Two things:
- Refined carbohydrates like rice, bread, pasta, and potatoes
- Sugar

In short, the Western diet.

Insulin Reduction

The standard model in the weight loss and health industry is to eat less and exercise more. Michelle Obama's school program, *Let's Move!*, is based on this idea.

Exercise is important but it's best when paired with insulin reduction. Insulin's main duty is to move glucose from the blood into cells to be used for energy or stored for future needs. Insulin resistance, the early indicator of prediabetes, prompts the beta cells of the pancreas to produce more and more of this hormone to keep blood glucose levels normal.

Gradually, pancreatic cells wear out, setting the stage for rising blood glucose, pre-diabetes, and diabetes.

Insulin is what's driving weight gain and driving chronic metabolic disease.

There is an answer. Reduce that sugar, and bring on the fiber. And that, my friend, is a snap shot of where you and I are heading.

INTERVIEW WITH ALUMNI
Linda Durland

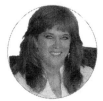

"It is not, 'I can't have that'. Instead, it's, 'I do not want that'. I am having to relearn who I am and who this person is—this thinner person." —Linda Durland

Linda Durland, 51, is a certified veterinary technician/office manager at a vet's office in Colorado. For fourteen years, this has been her dream job. She is married with a daughter, 19, and a son, 24. Linda grew up in Boulder but now enjoys rural Colorado. It's a slower paced life and everybody knows and watches out for one another.

When did you start 30 Days Sugar Free?
November 1st, 2013.

What kind of crazy thought was going through your head when you thought that was a good idea?
I really don't think I thought it through! I had no idea what to expect. I just knew I had to do something. I didn't have a clue but I didn't give it a second thought. I put myself in your hands.

What was going on with your sugar intake before you did 30 Days Sugar Free?
I ate sugar all the time—breakfast, lunch, dinner, snacks before bedtime, dessert. I didn't drink a lot of soda, but probably a couple

a week. The hardest time to eat well was when I got home from work and wanted to relax a bit. The first thing I would do was grab something to eat like chocolate—a handful of M&M's or a bowl of peanut butter.

For that first thirty days did you cut out all that stuff? Did you go totally clean?
I did! Certainly no soda or candy, not even a piece of gum.

What did friends and family say when they heard you were doing this? And as they watch you now?
For the first few months they just thought it was a fad or a phase I was going through and would say, "Oh, she cannot keep that up." I think my Mom is impressed but also shocked that I am doing this for so long. I had to tell her the other day, "Mom, this is my lifestyle now. It is not just a phase."

My M&M budget is down to zero—do you understand? Mom keeps telling me my butt is getting smaller so I guess that is progress.

Do people at work or in your daily life comment about it? How does it work socially?
Nobody really says anything, but I get reactions. I saw some people at the movie theater the other night that I have not seen in a while and I could tell that their eyes were going up and down. I could see the wheels turning like, "Oh, she looks like she has lost some weight." But they did not say anything.

My boss will occasionally ask, "How much weight have you lost now?" I think he is afraid to ask in case I go back to my old ways.

If you could take your mind back to the first thirty days, what was easier than you thought it would be?
I never had any craving or reaction like you described on Day 4. I never had any of those. I call that a God thing because to me that is just amazing. Each day was just like the one before.

Did you have any hard days? Or was it that you just stopped one day and it was never hard?

I was looking back through my journal. On a few of the days I had headaches but no battles. My key is I do not let myself get hungry and I always keep something handy that I can eat. Sure, I might *want* something else, but if I do not let myself get hungry that is what helps me power through.

I have noticed lately, though, that when I see sugar or candy or people eating that, I have this conscious moment when I think, "I could eat that—but why?" I have to have this dialogue in my head. It's maybe two or three seconds and I am not sure why I do it!

Was there any part of the thirty days that was harder than you thought it would be?
When I was in the thirty days, the countdown made it simple. "I have got three more weeks to go. I have got ten more days to go." It was all a mental game.

Once I got through the thirty days, it's now easy because it is my choice. I am not tied to being accountable to a commitment.

In my journal, I wrote that I have to tell myself: *It's not that I can't have something. Instead, it's I do not want that.* It's an old mental struggle when I am told I cannot have something. I am trying to reprogram my brain to *I do not want* instead of *I cannot have*. It's how I frame it. I have gone from *I cannot have this* to *I feel so much better when I eat this way.*

Beautiful distinction, Linda. What surprised you right off the bat about 30 Days Sugar Free and what has happened since then?
I can't believe it is now second nature! I do not even think about it and that is what keeps me going.

I do not want to have to do the 30 days again and it is a motivation for not getting started again.

Do you still feel that way? As of today you are just over six months sugar free. Do you feel like if you had something, you might be in danger of going back full-tilt?
Yes and no. I mean I still have not had any candy or cookies, you know, regular junk food kind of stuff. My version of sugar free is probably 95% sugar free, and it is mostly just the sneaky sugar and I am okay

with that. A tad in a sauce or a salad dressing. Maybe some in a piece of bread.

Is there any time that your body yells, "GET ME SUGAR!," or do you feel that has changed?

My relationship with food is so completely different. It used to be all I thought about—even when I was eating. What was I going to eat for the next meal?

Now, not only do I really not think ahead (unless it's about logistics to prepare), but I do not even think about really having a dessert or snack. Occasionally, I think I need to and then I just grab some raisins or something. It's like my whole brain has been retrained for the most part. It is easy for me to walk away from the stuff even when my family is eating it or when we go to Dairy Queen so they can have their ice cream.

I am thinking about something coming up. My son is getting married next summer and I have already decided that I am going to have some cake and be okay with that. I hope that is as far as it goes.

Nice! Could you spend a second or two talking about any changes you have noticed on the inside and outside?

Issues with my sinuses are starting to improve, so I am starting to sleep better.

Mental clarity has improved. I still get tired when I get home but nothing like I was. It's a different kind of tired. It is not like a drug-induced tired—it is just being physically exhausted. It's the kind of exhausted when you have been awake too many hours as opposed to *I have beaten my body into a poisonous death* kind of tired.

Did you see any weight loss during the thirty days and then in the past six months?

I think I lost thirteen pounds over the first 30 days. I weigh myself every ten days and that is what I have done consistently since I started. This has really worked for me because I forget about it and then go on with my life and then I know it is time to weigh again.

Right now, I am down 26 pounds from my sugar days! I had to go buy new clothes, so that was nice.

On a side note, I was really struggling with my new body. I have had help from my life coach getting used to this new body because I have been overweight for the majority of my life. I didn't know this new person.

I am having to relearn who I am and who this person is—this thinner person. I have gotten more accepting of it and it is not such an anxiety issue anymore.

I have been hiding behind my clothes. I am working through that. I am making progress.

CHAPTER 5
Types of Hunger

If you take away the fancy tablecloths and happy hours, food has one purpose: to provide nutrition and support us in living healthy lives. Here on planet earth, however, it's also used to show love, spare us from boredom, fend off loneliness, highlight celebrations, and dozens of additional reasons that keep food front and center.

All these are reasons why we eat, and each of them fit into one of two categories:

- Nutritional – We need it to live and grow.
- Emotional – Everything else!

In simpler times, food was used mostly for fuel so that we could have the needed energy to go out and hunt—for more food! Gone are the days of such simplicity around the act of eating.

In this chapter I look at a few of the ways and reasons that food is consumed in our modern world. I'm also going to use the lens of 30 Days Sugar Free to examine how these categories for eating can fit into the challenge you are contemplating.

Often it might seem that when you're really hungry, the most readily available foods are the quick and easy "empty" ones with little nutritional value. Perhaps there isn't time to cook a real meal and snack foods or fast foods are the quickest solution. Or you're feeling lazy—"Not ANOTHER meal to cook or plan for." After all, food and convenience are closely linked in our society. But if we don't fill up on good foods when we are hungry, a cycle begins. We feel hungry, we try to satisfy it immediately with a quick fix, then we are still hungry, we need to satiate the hunger, we go for a quick fix... etc.

How Food Is Used
True Hunger
Let's start with the simple one—we get hungry. While we have been programmed to eat three meals a day, it's important to remember that you have a choice every time you have a meal. Ask yourself, "How hungry am I and can I satisfy my nutritional needs without overeating?"

True hunger can easily become a slippery slope that lands you in the category of emotional eating.

Dehydration Hunger
Time for a 25-cent word: hypothalamus. Yep, that little part of the brain receives the message that you are hungry, and the wheels start turning. But guess what? Because of some not-so-highly-evolved design in your brain, the hypothalamus also receives the message that you are thirsty!

So how does a well-meaning person know the difference?

Often we use time of day for guidance. The three meals are fairly well placed and if we get the message and it's close to noon, we might just do the math and figure it's hunger. Safe bet.

But what about that same signal at 10AM or 10PM? 2PM or 2AM? Do you assume that dear hypothalamus is paging food or do you reach for something to quench the thirst?

Sugar Free Suggestion: In the chapter, *Food 101*, I challenged you to drink two glasses of water and wait 10 minutes before eating anything sweet. Now, I'd like to up the ante and ask you to take a glass of water and a five minute walk if it's not near meal time and you are feeling a pull towards the fridge.

Emotional Eating
The busier you are, the more important it is to have a way to cope with the changes, drama, schedules, and the emotions that arise from changing situations. One island of respite that is easily available is food.

Happy? Celebrate with something yummy! Sad? Grab something to ease the blow. Mad? That bag of chips is going down!

Sugar Free Suggestion: Before heading directly to the cupboard, take 5-10 slow, deep breaths. During those exhalations, experience the feelings that you are coping with. Beneath anger there is often sadness. While eating might cover the sadness, allowing yourself to stand in the fire of the sadness will ultimately lead to healing and stop the cycle that emotional eating perpetuates. Your feelings are the road map to healing—don't cover them in food! Adding a stomach ache to sadness isn't a win.

Emotional eating is a complicated topic and well beyond the scope of this book. If you feel you are suffering from compulsive emotional eating, please seek a support group or professional help.

Boredom

Browsing the cabinets or refrigerator for distractions from boredom is a luxury of the western world—and one we really can't afford. The costs of boredom eating are billions of dollars and thousands of lives, every year. With 70% of the American population overweight or obese—and on the rise—it's clear that we have lost our ability to regulate the partnership between our hand and mouth. By the time you're bored, it's too late to make a deal with yourself about eating. You've already tilted past the point of no return, and the feeding will surely happen.

I recommend paying particular attention to what you think and feel when you stand up to go eat because of boredom. Once you see a pattern, you'll be able to identify it well in advance and make a detour that is healthy.

Sugar Free Suggestion: Have "go-to" activities that you can lean on when those precursors to boredom eating show up. Walk around the block, do ten push-ups, drink two glasses of water—or come up with an idea that is personalized for you and your life. What a way to grab victory from the jaws of defeat!

Tired Hunger

Boy, do I see this in my 12-year old son. Come bedtime he will suddenly realize that he's "starving." He begins making negotiations worthy of a global leadership summit! After a glass of water and some conscious distraction—*Tell me your favorite part of the day*—he's in bed and asleep in less than five minutes.

Sugar Free Suggestion: Give yourself this time to slow down. Meditate, read, breathe deeply, or write in your journal. This might be a struggle the first few times. (Do I hear you saying, "Impossible"?) The call for food at this hour has nothing to do with hunger. Derailing the train en route to the pantry will make it easier the next time you do it.

Exercise or Hunger?

For many people, this is a very blurry line—especially if your work involves you sitting for long periods of time. These flesh envelopes we are wrapped in were really designed for movement. No position on the chart of evolution shows man in a chair slumped over a computer.

And sitting is a reality in our world. The challenge is to find ways to bring enough movement into your life that you are able to handle the sitting while maintaining a healthy body and mind.

Sugar Free Suggestion: Early morning exercise! Most mornings I'm in the pool by 5:30, at a cross training class at 6:15, on the bike trail as early as possible, or hiking my dog. I need to be finished with exercise by 7AM so I can be an active member of the family. Would you be willing to adjust your schedule to accommodate an early morning appointment with some form of movement? A walk or run before the world gets going is life-changing.

If that sounds crazy and you like me less after reading that last paragraph, then I'm going to suggest you modify your workday to allow for a 5-minute walk/stretch/push-up/plank or some other form of simple exercise each hour of your work day, and the aforementioned walk or run after work. Don't cheat yourself out of this experience during your 30 Days Sugar Free challenge.

Social Expectation

There are few things more bonding than sharing a meal with friends and family. The problems arise when it messes with your limits and boundaries. Being in touch with your fullness level might be easier when you are alone than when you are with company. Over-eating is a silent agreement people often have at parties, restaurants, or special events: "You don't point out the fact that I just ate enough for three people and I won't mention that you just ate enough for four."

Sugar Free Suggestion: Connect with your internal full/empty gauge. Experience the wonder of pushing a plate away when it is still holding food—or asking for a doggie bag. This little move is so empowering and will be noted by everyone at the table. Take the game even higher by owning your mouth and knowing when enough is enough.

Because Food is There

This is a 2nd cousin of boredom eating. It warrants mention here because temptation looms. Awareness and preparedness are your friends here. Instead of shoving a soda and hot dog into your face at a ballgame, bring a bottle of water and a piece of fruit. Simple. Effective.

Sugar Free Suggestion: If you are in the vicinity of a random feeding trough, limit yourself to one healthy choice. If there aren't any, use that time to socialize with others. Your empty hands will both baffle and inspire them. You'll also serve as a mirror where they will see something valuable in themselves.

Rubber Meeting the Road

Let's make this personal. Recall a time when you practiced one of the types of eating listed. To review:

- True Hunger
- Dehydration Hunger
- Emotional Eating
- Boredom
- Tired Hunger
- Exercise or Hunger?
- Social Expectation
- Because Food is There

Later in the challenge, we'll dig into habits and how to change them on a dime. For now, you are going to use an experience from your past to understand the triggers, execution, and outcome of your relationship to food and eating. This exercise will provide you with a schematic of how it happens so you can notice when it's coming and detour to happier ground. I suggest you write out the answers to help anchor the learning.

- When specifically did this type of hunger happen?
- Where were you?
- Why did you do the eating? (Choose from the list in *Types of Hunger.*)
- What did you eat?
- Who did you have to become to partake in the eating (an apathetic person, a lonely person, a desperate person, a sad person, an unconscious person, etc.)?
- How would you have wanted to deal with the emotion besides eating?

That's actually a very insightful exercise and I hope you do it. There will be magic and strength revealed to those who put in the work. There will be no benefit to those who don't.

You've chosen this period of time to look at your relationship to sugar. Essentially, you've created a laboratory for getting to know who you are around food. Don't sell yourself short by simply scarfing down a plate of whatever is handy. Research and record. You are worth it!

Recognizing Physical Hunger

Can you distinguish the differences between physical hunger and all of the other types of eating mentioned above?

The challenge I want to present to you is to consciously feel the differences and note them. Use this opportunity to do some testing so you can draw deep distinctions and recognize the control you have over your eating. For instance:

- What is the very first sign you have of physical hunger? Where is it in your body or mind?
- What happens to the sensation of physical hunger when you drink a full glass of water and wait 5 minutes?
- How does it feel when you satiate physical hunger by eating slowly? Put your utensils down between bites and chew each bite 5, 10, or 20 times.
- What happens if you eat until you are half-full and then walk away from the meal?

Remember the bigger picture I talked about at the beginning of this book? When others are eating just because food is there, this presents a big opportunity to model (for yourself and others) a new way of being. It's done silently, purposefully, and with great pride.

Mariella Kruger

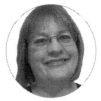

*"Going sugar free stabilized my mood to where I could
actually start dealing with some tough stuff in my life."*
—Mariella Kruger

Mariella Kruger is 48 years old and has two sons, ages 6 and 26.
She lives in Alaska and works as an administrator. She shares
her on/off journey with sugar free. She did the first 30 days and felt
great. Early into her second month, she decided she would dabble with
sugar and fell back into it for about five months. She went sugar free
again and I grabbed this interview when she was two months sugar
free.

Where were you with sugar in your life that led you to do this?
I've struggled with my weight pretty much my whole adult life but
especially in the last 10 years. I had tried different diets. I was feeling
a bit hopeless and then my brother told me about the 30 Days Sugar
Free challenge he was going to do. As soon as I saw it, I thought, this is
for me. So I just decided to do it.

**How would you rate your sugar intake right before you did it? Were
you heavily into sugar?**
I was into it really heavily. I would sit home alone in the evening
with nothing to do and I would start to get the sugar craving. Next

thing I knew, I was making fudge. I would just sit there and eat it. I wasn't even hungry. I felt the compulsion to have it. It was doing something for me. That was right before I started the 30 Days Sugar Free challenge.

So what did your friends and family say when you first mentioned it? Did you tell them you were doing it?
I did. It was not as difficult as it might have been right at first because my brother, his wife, and my sister all did it, too. They were pretty supportive during the first month.

My daughter-in-law was very supportive, too, but it was really hard on her because she would want to invite me over for meals like we had always done. She was very flustered about what she could feed me and had gotten mixed up with the nutritional information on labels rather than the ingredients. One night, she was almost in tears because she couldn't feed me anything. She was very frustrated. So we talked and I told her the difference. We had a really nice meal together. She realized it was doable.

She and my son have been very supportive. My son thinks I'm a little eccentric and he does tease me about not eating sugar. But overall, I view him as really supportive and he'll usually try something sugar free that I make.

Your initial journey was a while ago. Now you are sugar free for a record length of time in your adult life. What's been easier than you thought it would be?
Giving up soda pops. My soda of choice was Cherry Coke. I knew it wasn't a healthy thing to drink, but it had a real pull on me, probably even close to addiction the way that it would feel or the way that I would think about it. It wasn't just something to drink. It was, "I've got to have this."

I decided to frame it as, "I just don't drink it anymore." Then I don't have to fight with myself.

So that was a little easier than I thought. Sometimes I get a little squirrely and think, "Oh, I'd like a really nice cold Coke." Or one time I saw a picture somebody posted on Facebook of a Coke with ice in it. And I was thinking, "Ohhhh."

Are you a good cook? Was that something you enjoyed even before this?

My mom and my sister are phenomenal cooks and I was not the cook. I used to be a recipe-only person. I had to have a recipe, all the instructions, and all the exact ingredients. Otherwise, I couldn't make something.

About three or four years ago, I took some cooking classes from a plant-based lady where she showed how to make substitutions. Since then, I loved cooking. And I'm totally comfortable. If something has sugar in it, I just leave it out, or I substitute. This way of eating is great—you can make more of your own meals at home which is cheaper and healthier. So it's a win-win. The nice thing is that you know what you're eating and what you're putting in your body. There's nothing hidden.

What's a good example of that?

Pizza dough will typically have sugar in it, but I just add a little splash of apple juice.

Was anything harder than you thought it might be?

The initial change in how long it takes to figure out how to shop sugar free was hard, especially reading all the labels. I was frustrated at first and think that can put some people off. It seems that everything has sugar in it. So what can I eat? You have to give up brands that you've eaten for 20 years. You always get brand X and all of a sudden you realize, "Oh, brand X has sugar." You have to go find something else.

I'm so glad that I stuck with it because it does get easier. Now I know what to look for. I'm quicker at spotting the different sugar names on the labels. It's really not a problem now. But when I first started, it was a real bugaboo and seemed a little overwhelming.

Now I can go into the store and I just know what I get. I want to encourage people to hang in there because it does get easier.

Would you say it got to the point where it feels normal for you to be sugar free?

I think it mostly feels normal but occasionally an emotional feeling will still hit me. I tend to be an emotional eater. Recently, I was having a hard time and I got a very strong feeling that I needed to eat something sugary. I was able to calm myself down and I made the decision that the feeling of pleasure and relief I would get from eating something like that was just momentary. And what am I giving up in exchange for that? I'm giving up my stable mood, and I'm giving up my health. So why do it?

Were there surprises in going sugar free in other aspects of your life?

I think the biggest surprise I got was the easing of my depression. That was the most powerful because I've been plagued by depression for most of my adult life and probably a little before that—on and off antidepressants and doing counseling. The whole nine yards. And right before I started the original sugar free month, I was told that I really should go back on anti-depressants because I wasn't doing well. I could get to work, keep the house, and feed my child. But I was just barely maintaining.

I really didn't want to be on medication. They never work for very long. There are side effects. But then I started the sugar free thing and at the end of the 30 days, I did not have any more depression. It was kind of a miracle. I was not expecting that effect at all. When I dabbled and went back to sugar, I started feeling depressed again. They wanted to put me on medications. My counselor actually told me, "You need to either take the pills or go sugar free again."

My counselor had seen such a huge difference in me and so I told him, "I'll do it. I'll go sugar free again." I started again on March 5th and my depression is gone.

Also, I had been having a really hard time since my husband's death. He died back in 1991. During the 23 years since, I have had a horrible time getting through the grief process. That's a pretty extended grief period. I had so much trouble with it. And I've been sugar free now about 60 days or so. In the last three weeks, all of a sudden, I'm able to work on that and work through things—in a really big way. I'm moving forward with my life.

I've been seeing my counselor on and off for about 10 to 15 years so he knows me very well. Today, he actually said, "I don't believe that you would have done this well by now if you weren't sugar free." He said he has seen such a change in my stability of mood and my clarity of thought. He truly believes that getting rid of the sugar helped heal those things in me and cleared up my brain. It stabilized my mood to where I could actually start dealing with some of this stuff. He attributed a lot of it to the fact that I'm sugar free and I totally agree with him.

If you look at the first 30 days you could say, "Oh maybe that was a fluke." But when the depression came back when I was on sugar, and then, for a second time, eased away when I was off sugar, that's too specific to be just a coincidence.

Congratulations and I'm so happy for you. That's really powerful beyond words.
Yeah. I'm thrilled.

CHAPTER 6

The Hero's Journey of Sugar Free

Your life, just like every movie or play you've ever seen, has a story arc. From birth to death, we go through a series of initiations, challenges, defeats, and triumphs. Within life, there are many chapters. A rough outline might look something like this:

- Infant
- Student
- Adult
- Parent
- Professional
- Retiree
- Grandparent
- Death

Each of these chapters has a story arc of its own. A huge part of any story arc is that the central character (ah, you!) believes that he or she has the possibility of a big pay off at the end. One of the most classic story arcs is known as the Hero's Journey, and I want to offer a look at the 30 Days Sugar Free challenge through the lens of that time-tested arc.

The Hero's Journey (Very Abridged)

This mythological story structure can be found as far back as early Greek mythology and as recent as every blockbuster movie currently playing. Joseph Campbell, writer, mythologist, and lecturer, is credited with popularizing the modern understanding of the Hero's Journey. Below, I will summarize the stages and how they relate to not only the 30 Days Sugar Free, but also to making any changes you want in your life—inside and out.

The Call to Adventure

From a mundane situation of normality, some information is received that acts as a call to head off into the unknown.

This is what happens every single time we are faced with an opportunity to rise and play bigger: a new job, first-time parent, divorce, life-changing injury, 30 Days Sugar Free. The catalyst could come from an article, a phone call, something you see. You hear the call and know that it's one you must answer.

Refusal of the Call

This might be from a sense of duty or obligation, fear, insecurity, a sense of inadequacy, or any range of reasons that work to hold the person in his or her current circumstances.

The call that brought you to this book might have come from a doctor, a mirror in your bathroom, a comment from a stranger, or the wisdom that lives within. The refusal of the call might have shown up immediately, or maybe it hasn't come yet. It might be a voice that says, "I can't do this." Stay tuned. Sometimes it's subtle and often keeps you awake at night.

Supernatural Aid

Once the hero has committed to the quest, consciously or unconsciously, his guide and magical helper appears or becomes known.

You will meet several of these guides once you make the commitment. They will come out of the woodwork, the market, the internet, and even your own circle of friends. Someone will reveal the equivalent of a "secret handshake" and you'll understand that they are a part of your quest. (Note: this is my favorite part of the unfolding!)

The Crossing of the First Threshold

This is the point where the person actually crosses into the field of adventure, leaving the known limits of his or her world and venturing into an unknown and dangerous realm where the rules and limits are not known.

Can you feel this one in regards to sugar? Perhaps it's the first conscious meal; the first whole day; the first week. Each of us might mark the crossing differently; however, there will surely be an event, or moment, when you realize you are firmly on the journey to transformation.

Belly of the Whale

This represents the final separation from the hero's known world and self. By entering this stage, the person shows willingness to undergo a metamorphosis.

In the 30-Days Sugar Free challenge, this stage of the journey will surely take place in the company of friends or family and will involve something high-caloric and tempting or a comment by another that shakes your resolve. You'll hold tight, and others will see you as a person on the journey to transformation. That external recognition might or might not be mentioned aloud. Either way, it will leave a mark on most in attendance.

The Road of Trials

The road of trials is a series of tests, tasks, or ordeals that the person must undergo to begin the transformation. Often the person fails one or more of these tests.

This is where the story becomes rich and juicy. The tests, ordeals, and bargains with the visionary self—they all live here in this chapter. You'll be covertly aided by the advice of the supernatural helper whom you met earlier.

Apotheosis

This is a period of rest, peace, and fulfillment before the hero begins the return. Days pass and this way of eating and being feels easy or maybe more natural. Those around you might turn to you for advice on subjects they never have before. You might even begin to appear to them as a supernatural helper. (Hint: nothing at all is required from you to fulfill or even acknowledge this opening.)

The Ultimate Boon

The ultimate boon is the achievement of the quest. It is what the person went on the journey to get. All the previous steps serve to prepare and purify the person for this step.

It's day 30. Your mind is calm. Your weight is lower. Your skin is smoother. Every battle you fought in the last 30 days seems like a dream to you now. And the next step looms...

The Crossing of the Return Threshold

The trick in returning is to retain the wisdom gained on the quest, to integrate that wisdom into a human life, and then possibly figure out how to share the wisdom with the rest of the world.

Ah yes... coming back. The text you are reading right now represents what I did upon my return from the journey. What you don't see is the modeling for my young son that change is possible for anyone—a true hero's journey. Who is seeing you differently after this journey, and how will the ripples of your experience empower them? As you can see, the math becomes exponential.

Freedom to Live

Mastery leads to freedom from the fear of death, which in turn is the freedom to live. This is sometimes referred to as living in the moment, neither anticipating the future nor regretting the past.

And there it is in the final step of the journey. That Freedom to Live is the big pay off—inside and out!

After the realization of your own Hero's Journey, the new life you want is a matter of choosing and creating. You'll have the blueprint, and you will have already executed it with one of the most difficult subjects imaginable.

Jesse Lewis

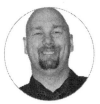

"It was a scary start because I really didn't think I could do it. But it's a heck of a lot easier than I thought it would be. Often, things are scary at first but overcoming our fears makes us play bigger in general." —Jesse Lewis

Jesse Lewis is a 29 year old hypnotist who travels extensively and works with clients throughout Canada. He has two children under 5 years old and he started 30 Days Sugar Free in March, 2014.

What was going on in your life like that made you think that this was a good idea?

I was sitting at 220 pounds, sore all the time, and couldn't sleep at night. I had digestive issues and constant heart burn. I thought, there's gotta be something in my diet that is causing this. I found out it was basically sugar. I had to change something.

That's fantastic. What did friends and family say when they heard about you doing this? What kind of reaction did you get?

Everybody said, "Jesse, do what you got to do. We've seen your health decline over the last five or six years... If you think this is going to work, good." Yet nobody wanted to do it with me.

It's not a sexy invitation!

This challenge showed me what could happen over the course of 30 days because I had a pretty drastic change when it actually happened. I lost 22 pounds.

Wow! That's really neat. What were you eating your first 29 years that you think was a big culprit and was it something that was hard to give up?

When I grew up, it was the '80s and there wasn't as much concern about a kid's diet. One of the things my mom did to get me to sleep was to put corn syrup in my bottle. It sounds disgusting but it would knock me right out. It's just sweet milk, right?

Apparently that translated into me really liking ketchup a lot and I would go through a bottle of ketchup a week. It's my favorite food on earth.

Oh. High fructose corn syrup and tomato paste.

Which is a lot of corn syrup going into your body. That was the hardest thing for me to give up. But after the first week sugar free, I found an alternative sugar free ketchup that tasted 99% like my brand ketchup that I used to go crazy for. And that was the only thing that I didn't eat completely sweetener free. I went to black coffee. I didn't use sweetener in anything else.

That's a really cool commitment for a guy on the road who moves around a lot. I know that's not easy.

I cooked food at home and took it on the road with me. But that only lasts about two days. I would find something in a small town grocery, like pasta, and cook it on the road somehow. Small town hotels—you don't have the best cooking facilities.

Was there any food that was easier than you thought it would be to give up?

I was able to find a lot of alternatives. There are processed foods that are sugar free here in Canada. Bacon was probably the hardest one to find. I did find a sugar and salt free bacon.

Was there anything that surprised you or you learned about yourself?

My knees used to hurt like a mother goose all the time. Once I went sugar free, a lot of the ache just stopped. During the time I was sugar free, I also injured my shoulder. It didn't hurt until I started introducing sugar back in. The pain came back and it was amazing to realize the reaction that my body was having to sugar.

Did the joint and the knee stuff clear up really early on?

I didn't realize how much of an effect it was having on me. I finally did get over that hump of not having sugar about a week and a half in, and I noticed nothing was hurting like it used to. I actually started exercising every day which is something I normally didn't do before that.

How did meals work with your family?

It worked out pretty well. I'm the one who cooks for the family. I was somewhat forcing them to eat sugar free food because I do all the cooking in my house. Sugar free doesn't mean that you have to eat plain bland food. I didn't realize that at the beginning because I can cook really well. I was trained as a cook for six years. I just never cooked without sugar before and finding alternatives to make things taste good was a big part of it.

I also thought it was going to cost more. In the end, I looked at my grocery bills and it was actually costing a bit less because I was eating at home more than anything else—not going out to eat and spending 50 to 60 bucks on a meal.

In the 30 Days Sugar Free, did it ever get to the point where it felt like normal? Like this is just what I do now or was every meal a thought?

It's the same as anything. Your first two weeks, they are going to be rough. Things are scary at first, but overcoming our fears makes us play bigger in general.

I love it. Did anything else feel different when you went off the sugar as far as sleep, anxieties, brain patterns?

Sleep was a big one. If I'm on sugar a lot, I cannot sleep. I'll sleep three hours a day. And when I'm off sugar, I sleep like a baby every night. The thing with my sleep is that when there is sugar in my diet, I can't stop thinking and it brings me down. When I went sugar free I was off pops (soda) which normally I drank before. I probably drank a liter a day. That could have affected my sleeping habits—too much caffeine.

And the digestive things—when I have a lot of sugar in my diet, I have to admit I am not regular. I almost had irritable bowel syndrome. Being off sugar, it made me regular. Within a half hour every day—the same time.

It's been about five months and you did six weeks sugar free and then started adding some back into your life. What was the process that led you to bring the sugar back into your life?

My basic process was that I could've sustained it if I was really, really focused on it—but with two little ones, and I'm their primary caregiver, it was tough. It was very hard for me to have their snacks ready all the time and not have sugar in them. When I was sugar free, I had a completely different shopping list for myself. There were probably ten items that were not filled with sugar on my family shopping list, whereas I had 40 or 50 items for myself throughout the entire month. It was hard to sustain, but more than that it was me being lazy.

And where does this fit in for a 29-year-old guy who has seen the change in his body and now he says, "I can't quite do it. I'm being lazy about doing it." What you are feeling and living with right now?

Looking at my actual meals, I eat now mostly at home and I cook most of my own meals. And most of them are still sugar free. It's the snacks that aren't sugar free. Like the cheese and crackers and things like that. I don't necessarily eat them myself but my kids do. And every once in a while, I will take it up. Like if there's a piece of cake, I may eat a piece of cake but it's not as often as it used to be. Now it's once a month.

So the drop in sugar consumption is probably about 60% to 80%.

That's huge. And soda, did you go back to pops ever?

I have a pop about once every 15 days. And I'll drink that thing and I'll think, "Oh, this thing is gross. Why am I drinking it?" and I'll switch back to water. So it works so good that way.

I also drank a lot of nasty juices. I learned the difference between good fruit juice and bad fruit juice. Many of them have a lot of sugar.

The corn syrup, again. I cut that out. I went down to water and juices I was making for myself.

Every once in a while, if I'm having a really bad day, I might have too much sugar. I know the next day that I had way too much sugar. I used to drink a lot when I was young and it's comparable to a hangover.

If could get the years back where I was young and being force-fed sugar by my parents, I would slap them and say, "Wake Up! You're programming me for life here!"

In closing, what would you say to somebody who was on the fence and thinking, "Maybe I should try this. This guy sounds a lot like me."
I think the biggest thing a person needs to know before they take this journey is that it's going to be beneficial—and to expect the unexpected.

The first week for me was horrid. I was a jerk because it was basically like a junkie coming down, right? But after that first week, I had a clarity of mind. My business became more productive. And it's a weird thing to see that sugar can change your relationships, but it can. If you are constantly moody, it helps. And you might not realize that taking sugar away can make you happier. It helps you get out there and do things. It can literally change your whole life.

PART II: HOW

CHAPTER 7
Preparing For Your New Habit

If you are at this point in the book and have decided you want to do 30 Days Sugar Free—YAHOO! The good news for you is that it all begins with that one decision. Since you've made it, the wheels are already turning. Drivers have started their engines.

Right now, you and I are going to lay some groundwork. Over the next two days, we are going to clean house and make sure you have the understanding and preparation to succeed. Two days is the amount of time I have found to be the ideal period between decision and beginning. It allows for the mental and emotional part of you to prepare, the physical part of you to get your ducks in a row, and the fight-or-flight reflex to be caught off guard.

NOTE: Eating sugar free will result in a healthier body, but if you are concerned about a specific medical issue, you should certainly consult your doctor before starting. I haven't seen anyone come out of this challenge worse off than they went in.

The Role of Sugar in Your Big Picture

There are only two times when sugar plays a major role in our physiology and behavior: when we are awake and when we are asleep. Aside from that, it really isn't a key player in the human experience.

In this chapter, we'll explore the cost and benefits of sugar in both of those states of consciousness. More importantly, you'll be better suited to connect the dots in your own life and have a more personal connection to the adage, "You are what you eat."

What's Your Sugar Story?

Everyone has a sugar story; where it fits in their life, how addicted they are or aren't, how they wish it was easier to control, or any of a dozen others.

As someone who coaches clients through 30 Days Sugar Free, I can tell you there are hundreds of ways people use sugar to hide, celebrate, relax, cover up, acknowledge, forget, or just plain drown out the noise and feelings of life. It's been the quick and easy cozy blanket to our emotions since we were infants. And believe it or not, for so many people, habit is the only reason they still eat junk food.

While I know there is a momentary peak that comes soon after the sugar hits your brain, the downside of it starts the second it hits the enamel of your teeth and continues on for the rest of your life by way of high blood pressure, excess weight, cardiovascular disease, depression, and a host of other ailments.

Quite the powerful negotiator that sugar, isn't it? I mean, if anywhere else in life you were offered a few seconds of enjoyment for a lifetime of collateral damage, you'd run, right?

For some, it's the moment sugar touches the tongue. For others it's the chewing. And another group can't wait for the swallow. Some get hooked on the quick burst of energy while others are all about the taste.

What I have learned is that sugary foods have a pleasure curve and a regret curve. For an overwhelming percentage of people, once the sugary treat is out of sight, the pleasure curve hits the ground and the regret curve begins its northern journey.

The Sugar Cycle

Regardless of where you find your particular enjoyment window from sugar, my surveys show that a few minutes after eating sugar, many people would love it if they could roll back the hands of time and get it out of their system.

Sadly, the latter can't happen and, to boot, it starts an insidious cycle:

- Racing heart
- Insulin levels spike
- Brain sends out dopamine
- Liver rushes to process the sugar into useless fat
- Teeth suffer the onslaught of plaque-causing chemistry
- Most ironic of all, the brain craves more sugar

Sugar is seductive and sneaky. Since birth we are bribed, rewarded, and punished with varying forms and amounts of the stuff.

"You've been such a good girl. Let's go get an ice cream!"

"You were a bad boy—no dessert for you tonight!"

Two of the first three ingredients in several of the most popular baby formulas are corn syrup (sugar) and sugar. It comes in early, trains the reward center of the brain to recognize and demand it, and, just like that, we are on the treadmill to becoming a statistic.

There's that sad statistic I've mentioned before: 43% of children and almost 70% of adults in America are overweight or obese.

Pass the donuts, please.

We Are What We Eat

In this chapter, however, we are talking about your new habits around food, so let me introduce a transition so abrupt, I might break a finger even typing it.

When we consciously choose to remove processed and refined sugar from our diet, we control how we feel, look, sleep, react, and ultimately affect the quality and length of our life.

Huge, right?

Exaggerated? Not even a little bit.

In today's global cafeteria of foods that include genetic modification, invasive pesticides, insane levels of added sugar, wine laced with antifreeze, pork dyed red to look like beef, and bleach-soaked chicken, "we are what we eat" has never been more true.

The majority of people figure that if it's in a box, a bag, or some teenager shoves it through the car window, it must be fine to eat. The fact that you're reading this means you are open to another possibility, especially as it relates to your happiness. So let's focus on that and see if you'll be willing to put your health where your mouth is.

Detoxifying In This Challenge

Many people have been addicted to sugar for as long as they can remember. There will be a natural period of detoxification for anyone doing this challenge. After about 20 days, most people say that the feelings of addiction are gone. Some people notice their cravings have stopped by the second week. From my experience of watching thousands of people do this challenge, the majority of them find that the chemical addiction is usually over after two weeks of no processed or refined sugar. Your body isn't demanding it like it was in the early days of detoxification. After that point, you'll be working mostly with habit, social pressures, and convenience.

The more water you drink, the higher your chance of clearing the addiction. I have a 1/2 gallon jar that I fill twice a day and keep on my desk. Drinking two of those is a gift to my skin, muscles, kidneys, and overall health.

Physiological Changes

There are several physiological changes one might experience during the challenge. Everybody is different and the experience is variable. Some common changes include increased energy and more restorative sleep, for starters. As your taste buds recalibrate, you will have greater awareness of tastes and smells. Some people crave more starch and protein at first, while some crave salt; it just depends. Your GI tract patterns might initially change as your body rids itself of the toxins it has built up from a sugar diet. This might include gassiness and bloating, but do not fear—it is a temporary side effect. People who experience headaches on a regular basis might feel an initial increase but notice a decrease as they continue into the challenge.

This is such a personal journey, and no two bodies will respond the same. That said, most people who go sugar free report an increase in energy and mental clarity, more restful sleep, and generally better health. However, during detoxification, the body might go through a host of changes. These are normal!

The Rollercoaster of Taste

Our taste buds are remarkable. Without you even thinking about it, those 10,000 or so sensory organs replace themselves every two weeks, and you can expect to notice a difference! What you have always tasted when you eat a food might be radically different once you remove sugar from your diet. Allow yourself a longer leash in terms of what foods you'll try. This is one of the most surprising benefits of stepping away from sugar for 30 days.

Of course, taste is a dance between the taste buds and olfactory sense. As an experiment, after a few weeks sugar free, hold your nose and try a food that you didn't use to like. This will isolate the taste buds to send the message to your brain for feedback. Many people doing this challenge are shocked to learn that they now enjoy foods that they previously couldn't stand.

Living and Eating with Others

If you live with others, one of your goals during this challenge is not to get kicked out of the house. This is your challenge, not theirs, and if you try and push it on them you are going to push them away. Instead, find ways to make it fun and give them ideas to help feel good about supporting you. Getting children involved in reading labels and knowing what's in the foods they eat is a skill that will serve them very well in life.

This challenge is a lot easier when the people you are living with are on the same page, but of course this rarely happens.

Know that change takes change. Most of the people that do this challenge have kids and spouses that are strongly entrenched in the standard, sugar-laden diet.

Having emotional support at home is helpful. Remain a clear example of who you are during this challenge and let them see your strength. Your family/housemates know what you're doing and dealing with it is really their work. You are doing yours. If they ask you about your sugar free challenge, be vulnerable and honest. Share the struggles and triumphs. That transparency is a welcome mat for them to share what they are feeling and experiencing.

Mindset Tips

Mindset is a huge piece of this experience. You've been coasting along how you have been for your entire life—and now you want to try something different. I offer these 10 tips in an effort to set you up for success. Give attention to these and see how you can incorporate each one into your challenge.

These are seeds you can plant right now and let blossom throughout the 30 Days Sugar Free.

1. **Define Sugar** – In this challenge we'll remove processed and refined sugars. We are aiming for the obvious culprits that have many names. You can find these in Appendix I: 50+ Names for Sugar at the back of the book.

2. **Share It** – Do you have a friend or two that wants to see you win? Tell them what you're doing! They don't have to be doing the challenge. This is about choosing a few people to "have your back" during the challenge.

3. **Get a Journal** – A journey worth living is a journey worth recording. A lot will come up. Write it down. You are going to be writing a best-selling book that is just for you. It will be there to help you in the hard times. Remember that very simple, but oh-so-powerful Lizard Brain? The act of writing takes your experience out of the unconscious, easily-forgettable place, and into memorable consciousness. I can't stress the importance of this enough—don't let the changes go unrecorded or unexamined. They are too valuable.

4. **Substitutions are Your Friend** – M&Ms become almonds. Coke becomes fruit-infused water. Cookies become apples. Get it? A lot more on this in the Daily Pages for the challenge.

5. **No Guilt. No Shame. Onward.** – Don't harp on what's happened. There is plenty to learn from any slips and you'll be well-cared for throughout the 30 day challenge.

6. **Enroll Others to Do it With You** – Is there someone you can think of that would be up for this challenge? Having both local and global support will give you the best chance of thriving each and every minute. Enroll them to do the challenge with you. They'll thank you at the end of the month.

7. **Reframe Your Negative Thoughts** – Negative: "I'll never be able to have a donut again!" "I will miss my _____ at night." When you reframe thoughts in the positive, your brain will be much happier. Positive: "I am going to bless my body and mind with 30 Days Sugar Free. I will improve my health by eating foods that support my health and by drinking a lot of water."

8. **Get In Touch With Your Own Higher Power** – that which you believe to be bigger than yourself. You are going to need both a mortal and spiritual hand to hold at different times in this challenge.

9. **Shopping List and Meal Ideas** – A starter list is in Appendix II: Shopping List at the back of this book. Modify it to make it yours and then carefully visit the store. Add to this anything that doesn't list sugar (under any of its 50+ names) on the label. Set aside some extra time to make new shopping habits, but I promise, it WILL get easier.

10. **Taper Off** – As you can tell, the practice of this challenge starts before you go sugar free. There is some planning and shopping to do. Some refrigerator and cupboard cleaning to tackle. Plan to start this challenge two days from now. Over these next two days, decline at least half (or more) of the opportunities you have to eat something with processed/refined sugar. This will make your Day 1 so much easier. Notice what it feels like to make that choice. Empowering? Easy? Extremely difficult? Use your journal to note what comes up for you as you simply pass on something you would have normally eaten.

Along the lines of that last tip: don't "stock up" on sugar in the days leading into your 30 Days Sugar Free challenge. I've heard from people who did this and it didn't serve them well. The fear that they will be without leads them to binge on sugar while it's still allowed. Tapering down as described above will deliver you to Day 1 in brilliant form.

The Most Important Meal of the Day

The morning meal is an important one in the 30 Days Sugar Free challenge, and here's why. The sugar level set in the morning becomes what the body wants to maintain all day. Keep it at zero. Ideally, you are looking for a breakfast that is high in protein. That is what the body needs in the morning so that it feels safe, cared for, nurtured. Not to say that there won't be some natural sweetness in the morning. I just warn against fruit smoothies or a cut-up fruit salad without adequate protein. While both are legal for the challenge, they will set a high sugar level in the blood that will be hard to maintain throughout the day.

It's easy to remember. Breakfast = Low Sugar and High Protein. The benefits of this wise culinary decision are many, and all of them have to do with keeping you healthy.

Protein:
- supports cell growth the entire day
- builds healthy skin, nails, cartilage, muscles, and blood
- does the grunt work of building/repairing our tissue
- produces essential enzymes and aids hormones
- makes you feel fuller for a longer period of time

By starting your day with a high-protein breakfast, you'll feel energized and ready to take on the day. I witness this firsthand on the days where I make my son a delicious two-egg cheese omelet instead of letting him grab a bowl of cereal. The differences are so easy to spot that even he admits it! On the other hand, if breakfast consists of a PopTart and a glass of orange juice, you are looking at a whopping 41 grams (or 10 teaspoons) of sugar. You'll set off the chain of physiological events described above, and there aren't a lot of ways to continue with grace after starting the day with that kind of smack to the head.

From a comment in a sugar free support group I lead:

"A friend recently suggested that I eat a protein breakfast instead of my usual porridge and the difference is remarkable. But strangely it has also cured my craving for sugar as the day goes on and I also no longer have the post lunch dip. Amazing."

Power to the people, my friend!

What About Lunch?

During the challenge, your body might play some tricks on you at the mid-point of the day. Look for the signs—headache, belly ache, inability to focus—and treat them all with the same prescription: two glasses of water. Seriously, drink them down before you do anything drastic. More often than not, hunger is a call for water and during this challenge you should never feel thirsty.

The mid-day meal is the most common meal eaten in restaurants. That's not surprising as most people are at work and have had enough eating out of brown bags during their school days.

The temptation to overeat unknown foods, unusual combinations, and sweet desserts is common at restaurants because it breaks up the day with something unexpected. A lunch break at work is a shining example of how food is often used for distraction first, and nutrition as an afterthought—if at all.

Fast food restaurants depend on people not to over-think their decisions. This is especially true in America where so many additional ingredients are added to make foods less healthy and more addictive. Examine this list of ingredients in McDonald's French Fries.

McDonald's French Fries Ingredients

United States	United Kingdom
Potatoes, Vegetable Oil (Canola Oil, Soybean Oil, Hydrogenated Soybean Oil, Natural Beef Flavor [Wheat and Milk Derivatives]*, Citric Acid [Preservative]), Dextrose, Sodium Acid Pyrophosphate (Maintain Color), Salt.	Potatoes, Vegetable Oil (Sunflower, Rapeseed), Dextrose (only added at beginning of the potato season).
Prepared in Vegetable Oil: Canola Oil, Corn Oil, Soybean Oil, Hydrogenated Soybean Oil with TBHQ and Citric Acid added to preserve freshness. Dimethylpolysiloxane added as an antifoaming agent.	
CONTAINS: WHEAT AND MILK *Natural beef flavor contains hydrolyzed wheat and hydrolyzed milk as starting ingredients.	
Source: McDonalds USA Website	Source: McDonalds UK Website

I don't know about you, but I really detest the thought of eating something that has 20 letters, I can't pronounce it, and is used as an antifoaming agent. Maybe you and I are just too picky!

Neither recipe makes me feel warm-and-fuzzy. I like French fries as much as the next guy but if I had to eat a bag, I'd hop a flight to London just to lessen the impact.

I'm not here to bash fast food establishments—people vote with their wallets and those places thrive regardless of the economic climate. The fact that you are here tells me that you are open to alternatives.

For lunch, just like at breakfast, we want to focus on protein and let that provide your body the nutrition and energy it needs. We'll do some fruit during lunch, too, to give your body the natural sugar it needs so that you'll have maximum energy and brain function. Choose a protein—meat, nuts, or legumes work—fresh veggies, some grains, and top it off with fresh fruit for dessert. Good parts of a successful day, right?

Dinner: Graze, Don't Gorge

One of the biggest changes for many people during the 30 Days Sugar Free challenge is that dinner doesn't need to knock the body unconscious for the night. It's nutrition, not therapy.

This is the meal where you have a real, tangible chance to move the needle on your body's big picture. What you do to your body during this meal is going to sit with you throughout the night. After dinner, there is often very little exercise, so your body has about four hours to deal with the mighty task of digestion and reconciliation.

Here are a few tips you can try that will yield a happy night for your body, mind, and spirit:

- Eat a light dinner. Smaller amounts of food make digestion much easier.
- Slow down your eating. Give your stomach time to let your brain and hand know you're full!
- Stay away from sugar. (No surprise there, I'm so predictable!) Anything you don't burn off ends up at the liver for processing. You know the closest and most convenient place for your liver to dump the fat? Your love handles!
- If you must drink with your meal, make sure you have some water. I'm not going to be the guy to tell you not to have wine or beer, or whatever libation floats your boat—just make sure you have some water. That, more than anything else when it comes to the end of a long day, is what your body needs most.

- Try not to eat too late or right before bed. Eating earlier allows time for digestion. Asking your body to sleep and digest at the same time is difficult multi-tasking.

In Chapter 9: Meal Ideas, I offer specific suggestions and leave it to you to mix/match to your liking.

Snacks and Drinks

I have conducted surveys with people who were considering a 30 Days Sugar Free challenge and without a doubt, snacks were the category of eating they feared most. Snacking happens for all kinds of reasons:

- Hunger (yeah... it's true!)
- Lack of proper nutrition during meals
- Stimulus – TV, billboards, smell of food, advertising
- Boredom
- Dehydration – I need water!
- Social eating
- Habit – It's been an hour – time to eat
- Transitional activity
- The introduction of a new or unusual food that "must be tried"
- Convenience
- See Food Diet – I see it, I eat it

One of the dangers of snacking is that it tends to lead to quick and easy foods—most of which are processed and loaded with ingredients you'd never consider eating if they were sitting alone in a bowl. Monosodium glutamate anyone? Don't mind if I do!

Often snacking is an unconscious behavior. During the 30 Days Sugar Free challenge we are aiming toward choice on everything that we eat. That alone will affect how you look and feel.

Drinks will include water, unsweetened coffee and tea, and diluted fruit juices.

Unsweetened alcoholic beverages such as gin, whiskey, and vodka are fine in moderation. Wine, especially dark reds, have less than 1g of residual sugar per glass.

Chapter 10 of this book is devoted to snacks and drinks. It's a big topic and I have got you covered.

Big Events

There is always going to be some event that will be occurring in the near future. Life is full of holidays, birthdays, weddings, anniversaries, and other celebrations. Many people believe they have to wait for 30 days free of these tempting events before beginning the challenge. Not going to happen unless you live in a closet!

Aside from your own wedding, I recommend starting as soon as possible. You will marvel at the willpower you will acquire during this challenge as sugar releases its clutches on you. I advise not cheating intentionally. Also, the word "cheating" is so loaded and you won't find it as a part of this challenge. You'll be asked to rise above habitual eating on a daily basis and a good wedding, birthday, anniversary, etc. is par for the course—and a perfect arena in which to challenge yourself to play bigger.

While at a special event, if possible, alert the host(s) that you have special dietary needs. If it's not possible, this is a good lesson in keeping some spare, perhaps homemade snacks with you at all times: trail mix, a piece of fruit, etc. When I first started my sugar free journey, this sounded strange and impossible. It quickly became very natural. Preparation is a huge key to success in this challenge.

Falling off the Wagon

If this happens, my first direction is, please, do not beat yourself up. I encourage you to share it with someone and then find what you can learn about yourself—and come back stronger! There is a huge amount of learning in this challenge and not all of it is about sugar!

You'll become more familiar with your triggers and how you handle them. In the past, that may have meant eating something sweet. Part of this challenge will mean "standing in the fire" and not covering your emotions with sugar.

Convert any guilt you have into power, and focus on moving forward. Reach out to someone and admit it—don't let it fester in the private part of your brain. The point in admitting guilt is to be accountable to yourself and keep it from turning into a secret that empowers the sugar habit.

CHAPTER 8
Preparing Your Kitchen

What Can I Eat?

Something I've heard from many people starting a 30 Days Sugar Free challenge is this: "What can I eat? Everything has sugar!" It looks that way, doesn't it? One of the 50+ names of sugar (see the list in Appendix I: 50+ Names for Sugar in the back of the book) can be found on the label for just about everything that comes in a box or bag. This wave started in the '70s when manufacturers were required to cut the amount of fat in foods and found a new best friend in sugar! As we continued to use our dollars to vote for what we'd like more of, sugar continued to be added to more and more foods.

Chances are that much of what's in your pantry and refrigerator contains some form of sugar. With two days to go until you begin your 30 Days Sugar Free challenge, we are going to change the landscape of your supply cabinets and get them looking like they belong to someone who loves themselves more than sugar.

It's Too Expensive!

One common objection I get from those considering the challenge is that "it's too expensive to eat healthy!" You'll find that you actually save money by not indulging in decadent, sugary desserts, sweetened beverages, and rich, sauce-laden entrees. Use the shopping list to stock up before starting the challenge. Depending on where you're starting from, you might already have enough of the basics in your cupboard.

You might also find yourself cooking more often rather than eating out, and this is a definite money-saver. I don't mean to overlook the time invested in healthier eating—that is certainly a "cost." It would be easy to say that you can't afford the time, and you'd be selling yourself short. Eating real foods is pretty simple once you get used to it. Give yourself a bit of leeway in terms of time and patience while you make the shift.

Taking Inventory

Go through your existing food supply and determine what from this collection you are going to be consuming for the next 30 days. To whatever extent possible, isolate your choices and keep them front and center. Pack these other foods away in boxes or simply choose a new area to store your sugar free foods.

Use Appendix II: Shopping List in the back of the book to create a list of what you'll use as your staples for these 30 days. While it may seem daunting at first, do this in small chunks. During the early stages, preparation is your greatest ally and improvisation is your arch enemy.

Create a menu for the first few days. You might have to grin and bear it and trust that you are doing something that is supporting the next chapter of your life. Enroll anyone you can who will support you, knowing full well that it's only 30 days.

Again—take this in chunks. For now, organize the first few days and allow your eyes to open into a new way of looking at what goes into your body.

Start With Vigilance

It takes vigilance, especially at first. Funions, Pringles, Doritos, Cracker Jacks… these are pretty easy to spot. Not so easy might be the $4 bag of Veggie Chips that look healthy. Example: A bag of Veggie Chips is not a healthy snack. It's not horrible, but for the most part your body isn't celebrating when it sees a 10-ounce onslaught of these coming down the pipe.

The Myth of Serving Size

"Serving Size" is arbitrary and might be two of the most ignored words on a label. It's used to juggle the required Nutrition Facts label so the food manufacturers don't scare the consumer half to death. That bag of Veggie Chips looks and feels like a healthy snack: moderate to low levels of calories, fat, sodium, protein, and sugar. Yet, on the label it is stated that this bag is 7 servings! I've personally seen kids eat an entire bag of these and immediately look up for what's coming next.

Contrary to popular application, neither the mouth nor any of the other six holes in our head were put there for the primary purpose of squelching fear, sadness, loneliness, boredom, or anger. Food is for nutrition and, percentage wise, very few of the 600,000 items that sit on the market shelves serve that purpose.

Truth in a 6 Point Font

They are ubiquitous. Sometimes small and hidden under a fold in the wrapper, sometimes proudly highlighted. The Nutrition Facts label is something that you have probably seen since you first started shopping and might have never truly understood. And they are often very small. If you're over 40 and anything like me, hopefully you have gotten used to taking your reading glasses into the store with you!

Nutrition Facts	
Serving Size 4 Bar (1g)	
Serving Per Container 4	
Amount Per Serving	
Calories 169	Calories from Fat 90
	% Daily Values*
Total Fat 8g	**12%**
Saturated Fat 5g	**25%**
Trans Fat 7g	
Cholesterol 5mg	**2%**
Sodium 15mg	**1%**
Total Carbohydrate 11g	**4%**
Dietary Fiber 4g	**16%**
Sugars 14g	
Protein 3g	**6%**
*Percent Daily Values are based on a 2,000 calorie diet.	

These labels first started appearing on packaged foods in 1986— and have been evolving ever since. They were originally added to educate people about the connection between diet and heart disease. Those were the days before 70% of the American population was considered overweight or obese. Today, those labels get a lot more eyeballs from people looking at calorie count and amount of salt, sugar, and other factors in controlling weight.

While those of us who aren't eating any processed or refined sugar tend to check the "Sugar" content on the label, that can be confusing. There are items, such as yogurt and milk, which will show sugar. However, that comes from the lactose. Since that is not an added or refined sugar, it's fine for this challenge.

Most items on the label list a "% Daily Values." Notice that there is no such number ascribed to sugar. Partly, this is because experts don't agree on the recommended daily dose of sugar. The World Health Organization recommends not exceeding 6 tsps (or 24g) of sugar for a healthy adult male per day. That would put items like most sodas, fast foods, and cookies in the range of over 200% Daily Values! Talk about a buzz kill!

One of the most overlooked numbers on the label is the "Serving Size." That number should really be considered first as every other amount or percentage listed on the label is per serving.

Ever see the amount of sugar or caffeine in a Monster Drink? The MegaMonster can is 24 ounces—3 servings! The can reads: Sugars – 27g. As bad as that sounds, that's nowhere near the real story. That 27g is for 1 serving. Do you know anybody who buys that can, pops it open, drinks 1/3 of it, and says, "Well, that's enough for now!"? It's a can, not a re-sealable container. The whole can is one serving for anyone wild enough to buy it. That means that 24 ounces later that person has consumed 81 grams of sugar! Let's translate that into reality.

Ingredient List vs. Nutritional Labeling

What if the nutritional label says 0g sugar, but there is sugar listed in the ingredients? Or conversely, the label says 10g, but there are no sugars listed in the ingredients. Which should you buy?

The short answer is that the ingredients list trumps the nutritional label. We put aside all foods that list any form of processed or refined sugar in the ingredients, but that does not mean we will eat zero natural sugar. Let's say that the nutritional label on a food reads 10g of sugar, but when you look at the ingredients, you see tomatoes, salt, lactose, and garlic. Some of the sugar is coming from the tomatoes (a natural source of sugar) and some is coming from lactose (a naturally-occurring sugar as opposed to a processed or refined sugar), so this is okay to eat. Other times a nutritional label says 0g sugar, but when you look at the ingredients, you see clover honey. Yes, honey is sugar, but there is such a small amount that there is not enough left after manufacturing to list.

Grams vs. Teaspoons

Do you know what a gram looks like? I sure don't. A neat trick to give sugar a tangible face is to divide the grams by 4. The answer you get is the number of teaspoons of sugar. That MegaMonster can we were talking about holds just over 20 teaspoons of sugar. Makes me wonder how many less people would buy that can if it showed a graphic of 20 teaspoons of sugar on the front?

If you are getting ready to try something new, check both the Nutrition Facts label and the Ingredients. If you see sugars listed in the Nutrition Facts, cross check it with the Ingredients to see where it's coming from.

Brands

The nutritional label and sugar content of an item are more important than its brand. That said, it can be difficult to find sugar free versions of your favorite foods, for example bread (or my favorite, sunflower butter). In the Shopping List, you'll find specific brands to prevent you from going on wild goose hunts.

Milk and Yogurt

This challenge rules out added processed or refined sugars and neither milk nor plain yogurt has any; rather they contain lactose, a naturally-occurring sugar. Check your brand of yogurt. You want to make sure it's clear of any form of added sugar. All flavored yogurts have sugar. You'll want to find a clean plain brand and add your own nuts and fruits. Milk and a list of probiotics should be the only ingredients on your yogurt label. No colors, flavors, sugars, or preservatives.

Breads, Pastas, and Potatoes

I'm often asked about these starches and the issue that they turn into sugars once ingested. This challenge prohibits added processed or refined sugars. As long as you choose whole grain breads and pastas that contain no added sugar, you may eat them. The goal is to get you through 30 days without eating processed or refined sugar. After you succeed in that, you can start omitting other carbohydrates from your diet if you wish. I suggest checking with a physician before doing that.

Honey and Maple Syrup

Yes, honey is sugar. But if you use a raw, organic honey, there is no added refined or processed sugar. This, by definition, meets the criteria for our challenge, and for most people, it is such a radical shift from their pre-challenge life. It's a loophole and one that you can personally decide to use, or not.

In the challenge, I'll talk about the taste of sweet and cravings. The idea is not to eliminate sweet tastes completely. We're giving our bodies a chance to recalibrate and have a new relationship with sweets. For some, any sweet taste, including fruits, will send them into craving more of that taste. For others, a small inclusion of a natural, unprocessed sugar will be fine. If you do feel the need, I recommended stretching a 1/4 cup of raw, organic honey or maple syrup over the entire 30 days.

However—and this is explained in more length when you are actually participating in the challenge—it is really up to you to decide your definition of sugar. Similarly, it is a personal decision as to what specifically you are going to pass up during this challenge. Some people will opt for no honey whatsoever; others will consider honey acceptable as a form of natural sugar.

Alternative Sweeteners

You are encouraged to stay away from alternative sweeteners during the 30 Days Sugar Free challenge. You are allowing your body to reset and find the natural sweetness that exists in certain foods. Alternative sweeteners tend to have their own addictive qualities, and their chemical-laden ingredients can do just as much damage to the body as sugar.

Sneaky Homes for Sugar

I want to tip off your sugar radar to these easy targets which you might otherwise miss. There are some foods that are just plain sneaky. Being ready for them will keep you from an early-game bobble. Below are the Top Five and some possible substitutions.

1. Ketchup – Instead, find a quality fresh salsa that's free of sugar. Tabasco sauce works if you like hot/spicy. Many members make their own sugar free ketchup. Check the Chapter 9: Meal Ideas page for a homemade ketchup recipe.

2. Mayonnaise – Traders Joe's has an organic brand that is sugar free. Most aren't.

3. Salad Dressings – Oil/vinegar is a safe bet if you mix it yourself. Also, Annie's and Trader Joe's make a Goddess Dressing—both are sugar free.

4. Sauces – just about every sauce you'll find contains some form of sugar. Use lemon juice, salsa, or mustard—and definitely ask your waiter to hold the sauces.

5. Dried Fruit – Check that label. Make sure you get it without added sugar. Ocean Spray Craisins, for instance, contain 29g in a 1/4 cup serving. Guess what? You just exceeded your recommended daily maximum intake of sugar.

A Happier Body

The happier you make your body, the happier you can be. You live in your flesh container and it is your responsibility to make sure it functions, hitch free, for as long as possible. We are naive if we think some charismatic leader, school administrator, or elected official is going to come along and fight the big money driving the food industry. It just isn't going to happen.

Food manufacturers are in the business of selling more food, and by adding sugar to everything from toothpaste to table salt, they keep us coming back for more.

Many people go through life eating as if all the studies and statistics apply only to other people. We wouldn't ever abuse our car the way we do our bodies.

My plea to you is that you look at all you have to live for—your family, your friends, your dreams—and you reconcile what you put into your body with what you want out of your life. We have a remarkable opportunity to control our health, weight, skin quality, sleep, anxiety, blood pressure, sexuality, and longevity. It dances with our ability to make smart choices about what we put in our mouth.

My invitation is to give yourself 30 Days Sugar Free so that you can be far enough away from the addiction, probably for the first time in your life, to design a new relationship with sugar. This relationship will serve who you want to be instead of who you are in the habit of being.

Give yourself the gift of conscious eating. You'll enjoy the rewards of that present for the rest of your life.

CHAPTER 9
Meal Ideas

Over the next 30 Days Sugar Free, you are going to have the opportunity to eat approximately:

· 30 Breakfasts
· 30 Lunches
· 30 Dinners
· 60 or More Snacks

At the beginning, it might feel like you are free-falling into the great unknown.

While the choices might seem slim right now, I assure you that by the end of the challenge you'll be well-versed and able to whip out or hunt down meals that are delicious, nutritious, and sugar free.

This is far from a complete list of meals you can have during this challenge. Please spice up this list all you want to fit your own tastes and cooking level.

In this chapter, I discuss the main categories involved with breakfast, lunch, and dinner.

Then I take you through a sample week to help you get started with some specifics. At the end of the day, however, we are eating real foods. If in doubt, use this question as a hip-pocket litmus test: "Does this item contain an ingredient that is out of integrity with my 30 day challenge?"

You'll know the truth in your gut—trust yourself.

Breakfast Ideas

As mentioned in the last chapter, this is THE most important meal of the day. There are many alternatives to sugar-coated, carbohydrate-laden breakfast foods.

Oatmeal – Try cooked oats with any or all of the following supplements: cut-up fruits including strawberries, bananas, blueberries, raspberries, raisins. Nuts add protein so consider chopped almonds, walnuts, sunflower seeds, pumpkin seeds, or ground flaxseeds. Spice it up with cinnamon or nutmeg. Add plain yogurt (no sugar added: Nancy's, Strauss, Brown Cow, or other clean brand), or milk. Both these dairy products will show sugar in grams on the Nutrition Facts label. That is a natural sugar from lactose—legal on this challenge. Note: All fruits can be either fresh or dried.

Corn Puffs Cold Cereal – This gets tricky but there are a few choices. Similar to oatmeal, decorating this cereal with unsweetened toppings that provide texture, taste, and nutrition is key. A great, healthy base can be made with a bowl of Corn Puffs, Rice Puffs, or Puffed Millet. These are unsweetened cereals found in most health food stores. Stay away from granola as it is usually sweetened with some flavor of processed sugar unless you make it. Have you ever considered making your own granola? You get to customize it exactly for your tastes. It's delicious and you might never go back! Check the Member Area for recipes. http://ILoveMeMoreThanSugar.com

Eggs, Bacon, and Toast – What? You didn't think we were going to take away the good stuff, did you? There are a few caveats with this option and they are detailed below. Over the next 30 days, you are going to be careful about bread. I have found one brand that is totally legal on the challenge called Dave's Powerseed. It should be available at better grocery stores and health food co-ops.

As for bacon—there are a few brands that are cured without sugar including Wrights and Gwatney's. Sugar is used in curing meats to offset the harshness of salt. Cured meats are pretty salty by necessity (salt being used as a preservative). You can order the cleanest bacon in the world from US Wellness Meats. It's really worth the price if bacon is your happy place. I've also been told that Kroger Grocery Store might offer a few brands of bacon that is sugar free. You can check with a Whole Foods Market, Trader Joes', natural food co-op, high-end grocery store, or your favorite butcher shop. It is the exception to find a bacon without sugar—be vigilant in your inquiry.

Egg and Cheese Omelet – So simple to whip up and clean up. Knock 22 grams of protein into your system and start the day letting your body know that you are taking care of business. Add in some of the leftovers from last night's dinner to sweeten the deal. I'm no Wolfgang in the kitchen, but this entire experience takes me just over 3 minutes to prepare and it's bliss.

Bob's Mighty Tasty Hot Cereal – This tip might just be worth the price of admission! A delicious alternative to oatmeal, this is available at most health food co-ops or bigger grocery stores. Add more liquid than they suggest or make sure you use milk or yogurt if you follow the directions. It can dry up quickly and turn into a mortar-like consistency unless you are generous with the liquid. This one is gluten free if you are trying to cut down on that, too.

Toppings? Easy! Use any or all of the additives suggested for oatmeal and enjoy.

Pamela's Gluten Free Pancake and Waffle Mix – Most commercial mixes will have some shade of sugar, however I found one that makes the best pancakes or waffles I've ever tasted. It's a mix made by Pamela's and again, it's gluten free. We know what you're thinking, "What do I put on pancakes or waffles with syrup and whipped cream out of the game?"

Here are a few ideas that will keep everyone smiling:
1. Coconut oil with cinnamon, cardamom, a sprinkle of raw shredded coconut, and a dash of vanilla—YUMMY! It makes Mrs. Buttersworth slink out of the room.
2. Greek yogurt. Check labels—the only ingredients should be milk and handful of living yogurt cultures that are difficult to pronounce.
3. Want to go old school simple? Try some melted butter, cinnamon,

raisins, or sliced dates. After about two weeks into the challenge you won't believe that this is almost too sweet!

Immune Support Breakfast

This recipe was offered from a member of an online group of people doing 30 Days Sugar Free. I tried it and loved it.

When purchasing ingredients, in all cases, fresh (especially organic) is preferred to frozen, and frozen is preferred to canned.

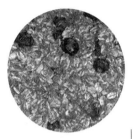

Combine all ingredients. Add enough liquid to cover ingredients and store in refrigerator. Soak the mixture for at least 30 minutes before eating. For liquid use water, soy milk, rice milk, nut milk, or fruit juice.

4 cups Rolled Grains:
Use 2 cups rolled oats plus 2 cups of some other available grain (rye or barley work well). Use 4 cups rolled oats if other grains are unavailable. Choose grains that are edible after soaking only. There is no cooking of the foods in this recipe.

2 cups Oat Bran (use rice bran if gluten-sensitive)

½ cup Fruits (fresh, dried, frozen) raisins, dates, blueberries, strawberries, etc. (without preservatives only)

1 cup Sunflower and/or Pumpkin Seeds (can be ground)

1 cup Nuts: raw, chopped, unsalted (I suggest walnuts and almonds.)

1 cup Lecithin Granules

*1 cup Ground Flax Seed **

*1 cup Milk Thistle Seeds * (Silybum marianum)*

½ cup Chia Seeds (optional) or Sesame Seeds

Spice to taste with coriander, fennel, and/or turmeric. Begin with 1 teaspoon of each. Other favorites include ginger, cinnamon, cardamom, nutmeg.

*Flax and milk thistle seeds are available at most health food stores. Grind them in a coffee grinder, blender, meat grinder, or mortar and pestle.

Lunch and Dinner Ideas

Lunch and dinner menus at restaurants have it all wrong. Often the menus offer the same dishes with 2 changes: price and serving size. In a healthier world, we wouldn't have a larger portion in the evening. We don't need more energy. We aren't starving. There is rarely anything that happens after dinner that supports the custom of eating more calories than we had for lunch.

What we eat at our meals should be based, to a large extent, on what we plan to do with the fuel we get from the food. If your post-dinner plans involve a reclining chair and a remote control, eat accordingly.

Protein rebuilds muscle and tissue as well as maintaining a more satiated feeling for a longer period of time. For lunch, while your friends and co-workers may end this meal in a self-induced food coma, you are going to fuel your brain and body with what it really wants. For dinner, think smaller portions as opposed to our cultural eating habits of large dinners.

Salads – You can have a field day with salads and the 30 Days Sugar Free challenge. If you have access to a place with a salad bar, you're going to want to hit this a few times each week. Steer clear of anything that you aren't sure about. For dressing, we suggest sticking to oil/vinegar—or pack your own Annie's Goddess with no added sugar. Most dressings have added sugar. Those listed in Appendix II: Shopping List do not. If you can include protein on the salad—like turkey, ham or tofu—you are going to score points for helping your energy level as you head back to the rest of your day. Also, add cottage cheese for a big hit of protein and good taste.

Soups – Not just for cold weather, soups are a perfect all-season lunch. Be on the lookout for soups that contain added sugar. This is a very good choice at a restaurant—a soup and salad will leave you energized, and without that post sugar drop that you know and (don't) love. There are so many varieties that I am going to leave you with these words—ask the waiter or read the label. The best choice is to make it yourself and there are hundreds of sugar free soup recipes online. See my favorite in the Member Area. http://ILoveMeMoreThanSugar.com

Sandwiches – That's right—we aren't robbing the backbone of the American diet. We are just modifying to fit the challenge. The main culprits here are the bread, cold cuts, and certain condiments. Dave's Powerseed bread is a good choice. Another alternative—Corn Thins from Real Foods. They are ideal for sandwiches because of their size, durability, and good taste. They are available at many grocery stores, health food stores, or on Amazon.

Protein

Yes, yes, and one more yes to protein. When your habitual inner-self is calling for a visit to the freezer or pantry so it can gorge on ice cream or cookies, it's protein and water that is going to step in and save you. The recommendation for daily protein intake is 46 grams/day for women, and 56 grams/day for men. Start early each day and drip it throughout the day for a steady stream of cell growth and repair.

Red Meat – For the carnivores among us, red meat offers never-ending possibilities for protein. From breakfast to dinner, you'll find simple and elaborate ways of enjoying the health benefits of beef, veal, bison, and other forms of red meat. Personal preference: grass fed, organic red meat. It's a bit more expensive and worth it.

Chicken or Turkey – If you're not a vegetarian, get to know the various ways to prepare foul as it will play a major role in your 30 Days Sugar Free. Loaded with protein, versatile, and not dependent on sugar to taste good, it will show up in various forms during your lunch and dinner options. Keep it as close to unprocessed as possible so you can know that it has not been prepared with sugar. For the most part, refuse sauces or any type that's flavored including savory, glazed, and barbeque. All of these will use some shade of sugar. A chicken breast often begs for some ketchup or other sauce. For this 30 day challenge, we are going to avoid ketchup and the like unless you make your own. Find a fresh, sugar free salsa and use liberally. Also, cooking with soy sauce or amino acids adds a delicious flavor.

Fish – Salmon, catfish, or shrimp offer dozens of possibilities for preparation and they are all very low on the mercury content scale.

Prepare by baking, grilling, pan fry, or steam. Each of these will give you the protein your body craves and is an excellent addition to the salad or pasta choices you have at your disposal. Tuna is another great fish option.

Salad, sandwich, or sugar free crackers—you'll get a protein rush (about 25 grams) that your body will enjoy from a can of tuna prepared with some (sugar free) mayonnaise, mustard, dressing, or straight from the envelope atop some celery, wrapped in a big leaf of romaine lettuce, or with an avocado. Many ways to dress this up include salt, pepper, dill, cayenne, or tomato.

Sushi – Stick with sashimi (pieces of fish with no rice) when possible, as the white rice in sushi often contains processed sugar that helps provide the stickiness needed to keep the piece together. You can order a bowl of steamed rice and sashimi and mix your own. There are also brands of unsweetened sticky rice you can buy such as Hinode brand, CalRose rice, and make your own. Also avoid fancy sauces, which definitely contain sugar. Use soy sauce with my preference—generous amounts of wasabi—and you're good to go!

Vegetarian Protein

Rice and Beans – With 7 grams of protein in a 1 cup serving, this is one of the best sources of protein around.

Legumes – This family of foods is vegetarian-friendly, versatile, and a clean source of protein. Good sources are peas (8g/cup), lentils (50g/cup), peanuts (35g).

Soy – Soy is a complete protein. Just watch out for processed varieties which often add sugar. Tofu, made from soy, is a good protein addition to stir fries and soups. The firmer the tofu, the higher the protein. At approximately 10g protein in 1/2 cup, it's a beneficial addition to your protein plan. Fry or bake it to lose the slippery texture. Then top it with salt, dill, or any other savory seasonings.

Eggs – One hardboiled egg packs 6 grams of protein. That, combined with the relative convenience, makes this a safe bet for the non-vegan in search of quick protein. Pack a few with a small bit of salt and you are good for an entire day—even without refrigeration.

Chia – Chia seeds contain 4 grams of protein per 2 tablespoons. They are great for making healthy puddings, thickening smoothies, or replacing eggs in vegan baking.

Seitan (Wheat Gluten) – All sorts of mock meats are made from this protein-rich food. Also called "wheat meat," it can be used in any recipe calling for the real thing. Check labels for sugar—my research shows about 50% are sugar free.

Quinoa – There are 8 grams of protein in a cooked cup and it is delicious. Add some soy or tamari sauce and mix it into the aforementioned egg/cheese omelet. Texture, taste, and protein. Winner!

Buckwheat – Its name is confusing, but this is not a type of wheat at all. It's a relative of rhubarb. Six grams per cup make it a good protein choice. It's traditionally made into soba noodles at Japanese restaurants, but you can use it as a flour or make the groats into an oatmeal-like cereal.

Vegetables

Let loose with your stir-frys, pan frying, steaming, and roasting. Think outside the box these 30 Days Sugar Free and reach to ones you don't normally eat. Jicama is a root vegetable that has a beautiful natural sweetness. Brussels sprouts and cabbage fried up in a bit of sesame oil with garlic will get you back in touch with the real flavor of foods. Steamed asparagus with your choice of sugar free toppings will put a smile on just about anyone's face, while artichokes hold their place as the dessert of the veggie world.

I'd also like give a tip-of-the-hat to greens. During this challenge you will benefit from foods that support cell growth. Collards, chard (check out all the great varieties), kale, and spinach will be honored guests in the eyes of your digestive system. Use the internet to find creative ways of preparing these important foods. Of course, you have all the basics, too. Have fun with the corn, carrots, broccoli, peas, and cauliflower—soon you'll taste a completely new sensation from these familiar standbys.

Starch

I'm not going to give these my highest recommendation due to the fact that the second starches hit your belly, they begin converting into sugar. That said, it isn't an added processed or refined sugar, so for the sake of this challenge, they are allowed. Exercise moderation with pasta, rice, potatoes, or breads—any of these empty carbs are not your top-shelf, go-to items for the next 30 days. Use them sparingly during lunch and/or dinner. Aim for no more than twice a day on anything from this group—and only once if you are interested in dropping pounds.

Condiments

Steer clear of most brands of mayonnaise. Duke's is sugar free and Trader Joe's has an organic mayonnaise that is sugar free. Relish and ketchup are sweetened and a lot of ketchups have high fructose corn syrup which is our nemesis this month!

You can make your own ketchup quite easily using a recipe from one of our alumni.

Blend together:

1 small can organic tomato sauce

1 can organic tomato paste

about 2 tsp vinegar

2 tablespoons of organic unsweetened applesauce

add onion powder, garlic powder, salt & pepper to taste.

This recipe yields a little over a cup of tangy goodness. Rule of thumb for ketchup—unless you make it, do something else—like a fresh sugar free salsa.

Dessert

This is the great wasteland for most people around lunch and dinner. It's usually not necessary physically or nutritionally, but the automatic habit monster grabs the fork or spoon and before we know it, we're wondering why we feel like crud.

> *"The meal isn't over when I'm full. The meal is over when I hate myself."* —**Louis CK, American Comedian**

Fruits

Fruit is an old school dessert. You remember my mini-rant on eating real food, right? Eat smaller amounts of various fruit for dessert and feel the wonder of how this fiber-rich sugar works with the body, instead of against it.

A Week of Lunches the Easy Way

One of the best ways to feel success is to prepare. I know I am reiterating this for the fifth, no tenth, heck, I don't know how many times, but it's THAT important. Doing what you've always done is going to get you the same results. Change takes change so consider this preparation for a week of sugar free lunches:

Sunday night: Slow sauté or grill a pan of red bell peppers, onions, eggplant, and zucchini (pick your favorites—this is my story!). Bake two chicken breasts that have been marinating in a bag of tamari sauce, ginger, and garlic for 12-24 hours. Cut up all this great (sugar free) food and put it in individual containers and store it in the fridge.

Monday: Mediterranean Wrap! Grab a tortilla wrap and spread it with goat cheese and hummus. Add some of the veggies and sliced chicken and call it a wrap. For dessert—grab a Fuji apple or a mango. You'll be the talk of the office.

Tuesday: Pick up a container of organic salad mix and add some of your veggies and chicken. Take your dressing with no sugar added. Add when the time is right. For dessert—some dried fruit or almond/raisin mix are delicious.

Wednesday: Do you do quinoa? This grain is fantastic and gluten free. You can cook up a cup and add it to some of your veggies, and maybe some chicken (if you're not sick of that calm, solid, steady feeling you have from Monday and Tuesday!), or just go vegetarian on this one. Use broccoli, chickpeas, and maybe some crushed almonds or pine nuts in there as well. Dessert for this one—how about mint or other flavor of herbal tea?

Thursday: Let's make a good-old-standby sandwich on a favorite sugar free bread, cracker, or Corn Thins. Stick with your chicken or other meat that isn't processed with sugar—there's really no need for meat to be laced with sugar. Lettuce, condiments of your liking, slice of cheese, and a tomato slice—and you are in control of what's going into your engine. Notice how you're feeling an hour later and see if the bread converting to sugar gives you a mid-day crash. Changing your diet is all about noticing the small benefits and consequences of your choices. Dessert for this meal? Get some healthy sugar that is packaged with its own fiber from a big juicy orange or cut up melon.

Friday: Your veggies and chicken are gone and you want to go out with friends, right? I knew that. Here are a few tips for restaurants to keep yourself running on happiness!

Stick with protein and real foods—that which had "eyes or roots" as I like to say. For dessert, don't get sucked into the instant gratification. Get a bowl of fresh fruit, a few dates with cream cheese, or a cup of tea. Pull off one week of lunches that look something like this and you are going to be shocked at how you feel and function. Treat your system like royalty and just watch who you become.

CHAPTER 10
Drinks and Snacks

Drinks

There has been noteworthy evolution in the human being over the history of our time on the planet, but it isn't happening fast enough to keep up with the amount of liquid sugar we pour into our bodies.

My son's dentist told him to not drink Gatorade unless he was actually holding a toothbrush! A 2006 study from the University of Iowa School of Dentistry shows that sports drinks erode teeth even faster than Coke and other sodas. The reported evils of soda include, but are not limited to: heart attack, high blood pressure, stroke, osteoporosis, type 2 diabetes, fatty liver disease, liver failure, and of course, obesity.

All of this begs the question: what can we drink that is good for the body and quenching to the throat.

My suggestions here come with the caveat that change takes change, and none of this is going to offer the same level of satisfaction right off the bat. As I've mentioned, but perhaps in different words, you're going to have to want the benefits of sugar free more than you want the immediate satisfaction that sugar-laden foods offer. It's a balancing act.

"What would you like to drink?" is a question that can be heard at just about every transitional point in the day. In this section, I'll offer suggestions on how to answer that question in a way that supports your 30 Days Sugar Free path.

Water – Your best friend during this challenge is going to be water. Lots of water. I know this came up a number of times in the book. Unsexy as it is, this 30 days is a detox and there is nothing better for moving the sugar and toxins out on a constant, dependable frequency. Try drinking water when you think you are hungry. Often dehydration manifests itself in feelings of hunger, but it is really water that your body is craving, not food. You will want to drink water at least every fifteen minutes while you are awake—keep a refillable bottle handy. You want to make it easier on your body during this period of detox. If you feel thirsty, you waited too long to drink.

Coffee – I realize that I might be treading on shaky ground here, but have your coffee without any sweetener. There, I said it—and I can hear your reaction! Let your taste buds begin to recalibrate. Even cut back to a smaller cup if that's what it takes. The relationship between humans and coffee is ancient. It's part ritual, part habit, part bliss. This 30 Days Sugar Free is an opportunity to experience coffee in a whole new way. Many 30 Days Sugar Free folks have found that a bit of cinnamon works really well in coffee.

Tea – If you can, get organic. Fruit, herbal, black, green, or white—your taste buds are going to come around and find what you might have always missed. Put two tea bags of fruit or herbal tea in a Mason glass canning jar and set in the sun for an hour. Then add a splash of fruit juice.

Fruit Juice – Fruit juices are acceptable during the 30 days. However, I recommend diluting the juices with water; usually a 4:1 water to juice ratio is fine, but certain juices should be diluted more. The cherry and mango nectar from Trader Joe's, for instance, are intense and can be diluted to a 10:1 water to juice ratio. I am also a big fan of squeezing a lemon, lime, or orange into a pitcher of water and have it available. Cucumber and melon also make wonderful infusions. Add juice to iced tea or a flavor-free sparkling water for an extra fizzle.

Milk – Diary milk contains lactose, a naturally-occurring sugar. For the purpose of the challenge, sugar is not added so it is acceptable. Milk from other sources such as almond, rice, soy, and hemp are processed and many contain some form of added sugar. Check that label for sugar in the ingredients.

Smoothies – Have you noticed that frozen fruit often tastes so much sweeter than its room-temperature counterpart? Let's use that bit of chemistry to our advantage!

Frozen mango, banana, blueberries, some milk, ice, and sugar-free protein powder create a sweet delight and will naturally satisfy the call for sugar. I suggest making your own smoothies whenever possible as you'll know what goes into them. If you order one out in the world, tell them to please stick to real ingredients—fruit, milk, ice. They often include sweetened powders and squirts of mystery liquid—no thanks!

Alcohol – You can drink alcohol which contains no added sugar. The grapes used for wine have a high sugar content (mostly fructose) and that is exactly what ferments into alcohol. Therefore, the resulting wine itself has very little residual sugar—often less than a gram per liter! Dry reds usually have less than light reds or white wine. Be sparing with it, or commit to the 30 days without. Hard liquors are case-by-case. Vodka, gin, rum, whiskey, and tequila (100% de agave) are sugar free. Most likely, if they are flavored, they contain sugar. Mixers—forget them. It's 30 days—you can do this and the rewards are so worth it!

Snacks

Treat yourself like someone you love and deeply care for and you'll instantly begin to reap the benefits of your efforts. To do 30 Days Sugar Free you'll be responsible for every bite you take. Hint: carry a small cooler with a few containers of mini carrots, almonds, cheese sticks, fruit, and lots of water. You know, real food? I guarantee you that packing all that into a small cooler will cost you less than a $4 bag of chips, and your body will thrive on such snacks.

I'm going to put my fingers in my ears and sing nonsense if you tell me you don't have time to prepare snacks for the day. That cooler will take you about three minutes to pack. (That's less time than it takes to get through a McDonald's drive thru!) Between the money you'll save, the peace of mind that comes from knowing what you're eating, and how good you'll feel—the time you spend will pay generous dividends—immediately and for the rest of your life.

You are going to figure out what works for you including how much and how often. Here are some suggestions that have been passed around our 30 Days Sugar Free community. Know that the first few days are going to be a challenge and you'll really have to be on top of yourself. You might have spent most of your life eating without much conscious awareness around ingredients—and you've chosen this time to make a change.

Sunflower Seeds – Eat these whole or shelled.

Nuts/Legumes – Almonds, peanuts, walnuts, cashews, pistachios, lentils, etc.

Fruit – Eat fresh or dried. Use these liberally during the 30 Days Sugar Free. Fruit will give you energy and is loaded with fiber which helps the body slowly absorb and use the natural sugar.

Ants in the Tree – This is a fancy name for celery with peanut butter and raisins.

Chips and Salsa or Guacamole – Make it yourself or make sure it's sugar free.

Jerky – Beef, turkey—make it yourself with a dehydrator. Most commercially produced jerky that you buy is loaded with sugar. To make it yourself: cut the meat very thin, marinate overnight in a ziplock baggy filled with tamari, ginger, and garlic, and then dehydrate.

Corn Thins by Real Foods – Top with some cheese, veggies, hummus, or nut butters (with no added sugar).

Use the ideas in this section—along with your own creativity—to get through the early days of the challenge. After a week you'll have a very good idea of what you are choosing to eat for this challenge.

Here We Go

In the first part of this book I've shared everything I've learned through personal experience, interviewing experts, coaching others, and extensive study about successfully navigating 30 Days Sugar Free. It's impossible to calculate how much more you know about the topic right now than I knew back on Leap Day 2012 when I decided to give it a try! I hope you'll apply all of it to succeed in a challenge that will certainly teach you a lot about yourself.

When you've prepared yourself for success, turn the page and begin on Day 1. Find a time to read each daily page and keep it consistent for the 30 Days Sugar Free. While doing this is completely your decision, know that there are people around the world who have walked the path and are cheering you on.

PART III:
THE CHALLENGE

Daily Pages

The Daily Pages are designed to be read, wait for it… daily! There is no reason to skip ahead as each day contains what I'd like you to hold in your heart and mind for that day.

Each one offers some combination of perspective, coaching, recipes, reminders, engagement ideas, and certainly a few words about how I am in awe of you for doing this challenge. Visit the Daily Page first thing in the morning if possible, when your mind is most open to suggestions. I trust you'll find something in each and every one that helps you over a bump in that day's road.

On some of the days you will be asked to journal. Do it.

On other days I ask you to go to the Member Area for additional support via a video, audio, or written supplement. Do it.

It is important to keep track of your experiences during this challenge as that collection of insights and revelations will be your best friend in the hard moments that will show up. If you have difficulty writing in an actual notebook or journal, I urge you to use a computer. If typing is another deterrent, you can use a speech to text feature on your computer or smart phone.

We are literally messing with the DNA over these 30 Days Sugar Free, and the more connected you are to yourself, the more centered you will be throughout the transition. That journal will act as a beacon during this 30 Days Sugar Free—and for years to come. If you are expecting to track your progress just in your head, you'll never recognize the changes. A lot of your brain doesn't want this change, and it will mess with your memory and results. Access to a journal of feelings, thoughts, and a life clear of sugar will give you a valuable perspective of who you are.

Thirty days is plenty of time to develop a new habit. One of the joys for people doing this challenge is the first day they go morning to night without a fight. I look forward to you enjoying that moment.

The more you put into this challenge, the more you'll get out of it. Trust the process and bask in the new reality you are about to create.

DAY 1
Stepping Onto
The Path

The journey of 30 Days begins with the first day—and here you are. I am so proud of you for taking this step. I'm guessing that your decision to do this challenge didn't make you the most popular person at the party. You might have even come up against some harsh questioning, warnings, or confrontations from friends or family. Relax, I'm not psychic. I've been there and heard plenty of it aimed at myself or clients over the years.

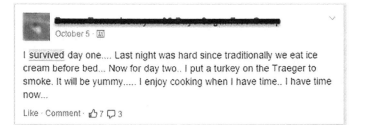

October 5 · 🄰

I survived day one.... Last night was hard since traditionally we eat ice cream before bed... Now for day two.. I put a turkey on the Traeger to smoke. It will be yummy..... I enjoy cooking when I have time.. I have time now...

Like · Comment · 👍 7 💬 3

This is the day when you step onto the path and make some choices that look different than what you're used to making. Certainly different than most people around you are making. It's a day to behold the peaceful warrior in you—the part that doesn't shrink away from the challenge and is unwavering in the mission.

The habit of picking up food without considering the ingredients comes so naturally. Perhaps for the first time in your life, you are deeply aware of what you put into your body. Take great care of yourself today.

Coaching

With yourself and with others, compassion will be key. Your brain knows what you're up to. It got the message from your heart about how badly you want this. What happened when your brain got the message? It probably snickered, or flat out laughed.

Whether or not you heard the chuckle, for thousands of years mankind has feared and resisted. It's an old reflex—nothing you are personally in charge of correcting. What we are going to do is work with that part of the brain. We are going to let it know that you are safe. You are doing this 30 Days Sugar Free to take care of yourself. More on that over the next few days.

Journal

I suggest that you keep some written record of what you eat. You can write it into your journal or a computer document. Put everything down—meals, snacks, drinks, quantities. How different is it for you to record what you eat? Hopefully it's very different! Shaking up the routines around food is something we are going to do a lot of during this 30 Days Sugar Free.

Oh, and while you have that journal out, jot down a few notes in response to the following prompts:

- Fears
- Excitement
- Any physical observations
- What brought you here? Weight loss? Personal challenge? Overall health?
- What do you believe the prize will be for doing it, and what might be the cost if you don't?

Courage and Resilience

Can you muster up extra doses of courage and resilience in yourself today? Both qualities will serve you well as you face your typical daily activities with these attributes.

- Courage to see the bigger version of yourself that goes to sleep tonight with a sugar free day in the log book.
- Resilience to recover quickly from feelings of loss, deprivation, or limits.

Know that this challenge is for 30 days and will give you insights that will serve you for the rest of your life.

Protein

Start your day with protein. The sugar level set in the morning becomes what the body wants to maintain all day so keep it low. A bowl of oatmeal or other warm cereal with a few almonds, raisins, and banana slices will give you 25% of your suggested daily protein. Eat more slowly than usual and take the time to actually chew your food—10 or more chews per bite.

Engagement

Over the course of the next 30 days I am going to ask you to get out of your comfort zone. Some of my requests will be easy-peasy. Others might have you rolling your eyes and wondering what you're doing here.

The invitation is to stay here through all of it. Allow me, if you will, to drive the bus during these daily meetings. Know that the moments in which you are least comfortable offer the greatest opportunity for change. If this were easy, you'd already be doing it.

I'll see you tomorrow. Enjoy the sweetness of the day in places that you might not normally look.

Your Personal Why List

Y ou made it through Day 1—Fantastic! Just writing that brings up early memories from my Day 2. All the empowering thoughts I had waking up for that 2nd day:

- how easy this is
- why haven't I always been sugar free?
- I've got this in the bag!
- I feel fantastic!

You know, the glow of the honeymoon in all its beauty; the wisdom and clarity of a 12-year old on that day s/he wakes up and realizes that they know and understand everything! Hearty congratulations for grabbing the looking glass and being conscious of what you are taking in. It might get a bit harder, and then a whole lot easier. My hope is that you got through Day 1 just by hook or by crook. You grabbed the opportunity to look at the big culprits, realized what you've been eating, and how it feels to turn away. Now that you have successfully made it through Day 1—let's do something together.

Journal

Do you have a journal or one place where you are recording your experiences over these 30 days? Please say, "Yes!" It's important as that collection will be your best friend in the hard moments that will show up.

Let's examine a few prompts:

1. The reason I am doing this 30 Days Sugar Free is...
2. What I think I'll learn about myself is...
3. What I'm afraid I'll learn about myself is...
4. The clear list of what I will put aside for these 30 days is...
5. The foods that will give me sweetness over these 30 days are...
6. This is what completing 30 Days Sugar Free means to me...
7. The best part of that will be...

Spend at least 15 minutes on these. The easy answers will come first, and the far more interesting answers are closer to the center of the onion—so take some time and peel it.

I'm asking you to do this because while willpower, novelty, and determination carried you breezily through yesterday, there is a bit of a battlefield on the horizon. The writing you do with these prompts will be your ally—and very welcome.

Change takes change.

If it's uncomfortable for you to write some of these answers—excellent. Embrace the opportunity to challenge yourself and stay in the game. Distractions will call you—that's a given.

In a few days, I will share my answers to these prompts. It's important that you have time to be with the prompts without going right to reading someone else's. That, as you might imagine, would be a distraction from doing the work.

Coaching

The word for today is novice—a person new to or inexperienced in a field or situation.

You have been you for a very long time. You are an expert at being you. Unbelievable at being you, actually. No one is better.

For these next 30 days, you are taking one of your most basic needs—eating—and laying it out on the table for examination. You are new and inexperienced at this, and on this second day, it's important to acknowledge that you are a novice. Give yourself permission not to know everything that's happening.

What else is there in your life that you do every single day at which you can say you are a novice?

Be kind with yourself. A slip up isn't the end of the world. Not knowing the answer, the next move, or even what you feel is expected. Can you hold the unknowing as a gift?

In this challenge, you're not the expert at being you that you normally are :)

Digging Deeper

There's a book I recommend to you at this early stage of the game. It's called *The War of Art* by Steven Pressfield.

In this book of short essays, the author shares the experiences of the protagonist whose name is Resistance. It applies to exactly what you are doing here. The short pieces in that book might just give you answers or insights into questions that you have been asking yourself about behaviors or habits.

This book hasn't been out of my backpack in two years and I open it constantly for reminders, prompts, or a perspective that is typically more on target than "the story" I'm convinced is true.

There is a link to this book in the Member Area.
http://ILoveMeMoreThanSugar.com

Engagement

Dig under your story of food and sugar in search of a deeper truth about yourself. To that end I am asking you to do some writing in reaction to those prompts. Some of those prompts require the left/analytical side of the brain, and others will tap into the right/emotional side of the brain. Not accidentally, the questions are mixed up so as to fully integrate the whole brain throughout the writing.

At this early juncture, I want to plant an idea with you and see if it takes root. Over the next 30 days, the idea is to discover new sensations of taste and relationships to food. I could easily create substitution tables that will leave you saying, "This isn't as good as the original," and that would be a disservice to you.

The invitation right now is to explore this big 'ol world of ours and see what foods and tastes have been hiding. What can you discover in iced tea with an orange squeezed into the pitcher? How could 12 dates, soaked for an hour in 1/2 cup of hot water and then food processed to a puree, replace refined sugar in anything you cook? Where has the delicious sweetness of celery, peanut butter, and a few raisins been hiding your whole life?

I'll fill the daily pages with some great ideas and recipes over the next four weeks. Today, however, my novice friends, I ask you to rediscover something that has natural sweetness.

In a few weeks, your taste buds are going to be alive and popping and even a Fuji apple might send you over the edge!

Move forward into Day 2 with compassion for yourself and those you encounter.

I'm Bored...
What Can I Eat?

When you go to sleep tonight this challenge will be 10% complete—how cool is that?

> October 3 · 🅰
>
> Day 3......Amazing. I feel amazing, more energy, less pain, no swelling in my feet, no sugar in my diet!!!!!
> Thank you Barry, Michelle and ███████████████ for helping and guiding me through this process!!!!
>
> Unlike · Comment · 👍 9 💬 3

First off—I want to check in with you about the writing prompts from Day 2. Did you spend some time on them? It's really important that you peel back a few layers of the onion as to the "Big Why" surrounding these 30 days, and here's the reason.

Here on Day 3, the voices of habit and sugar might start getting a bit louder and success will depend upon you having some emotional connection to the reasons you're doing this. Please—go do it now if you haven't already.

If you did respond to the prompts, congratulations and keep the journal handy. In the trying moments, open it up and fill yourself with those sobering words you wrote.

The parts of you that need to step up will thank you.

Snacks

There is always the issue of snacks. That was also the #1 reply to our survey when I asked the online community, "Which do you think is the most challenging time of the day?"

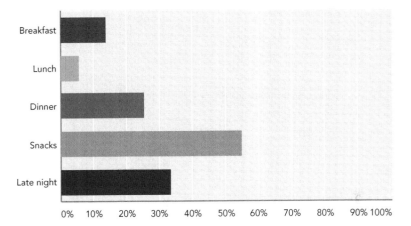

Favorites

Let's take a look at some of the favorite sugar free snacks from those that have completed this challenge. The key to snacks is to be prepared. Some of these snacks should be on your person at all times, just in case. See Chapter 9: Meal Ideas for more sugar free snacks.

1. **Trail Mix** – Make it yourself or pre-made. Watch out for chocolate, yogurt chips, or sugared dry fruit, which are often added to the store-bought varieties.

2. **Dried Fruit** – Mango, apricot, raisins, strawberries, bananas – Trader Joe's or your local health food store have great selections. Make sure you buy the kind that isn't sugar-coated or sprayed with sulphur dioxide. There's absolutely no reason to eat those additives.

3. **Apple Slices with Nut Butter** – Almond, peanut, sunflower, cashew—get the ones without any added sugar (watch out for "evaporated cane juice" on the label). This is a hearty and healthy snack, as well as a great source of fiber and protein.

4. **Popcorn** – Add nutritional yeast to the top and enjoy. More topping ideas? Dill, cinnamon, lemongrass, cayenne pepper, Parmesan cheese, and of course, butter and salt.

5. **Avocado with a Dash of Salt** – Enough said, right? Depending on your tastes and desires, use some tomato, lemon, or cayenne pepper to season this wonderfully healthy treat.

Coaching

As you move through your day, make visual contact with a food that you would have normally picked up and chomped down. This includes the unconscious ones that come across your path and you pick up for comfort, to satisfy a social expectation, or just out of habit. Habit and comfort are discussed in the chapter, *Living in the Habit.*

The challenge is to hold that visual contact for a full 15 seconds and take three very slow, deep breaths. Observe what is happening in your body during those breaths and come out of the gaze with one word in each of these three categories:

· Physical Feeling (examples: Grab, Bite, Lick, Suck, Chew)
· Emotional Feeling (examples: Mad, Sad, Glad, Scared, Ashamed)
· What I Feel From Walking Away (examples: Strong, Proud, Controlled, Beautiful, Confident)

Three words.
Let those roll around in your mind while you take three slow, deep breaths.

Journal

Write those three words in your journal—and make them bold. Have fun with the letters and words. These words have to be memorable to both the conscious and unconscious mind.

Do this with at least two other food products.

If you happen to be in a market, you can do it three times in one fell swoop. What about doing this with cookies, flavored yogurt (which is basically melted ice cream), and soda?

Engagement

There is a scene from the TV series, *Seinfeld*, where George realizes that "every decision I've ever made in my life was wrong!" It's a classic scene that shows what might happen if we do the opposite of what we've always done. I think it aligns perfectly with the mission for this challenge on Day 3. Watch it in the Member Area for Day 3. http://ILoveMeMoreThanSugar.com

See you on Day 4!

DAY 4
Ground Zero

This is a very personal day in my 30 Days Sugar Free history book. I remember very clearly sitting on my couch and for some reason, I was holding this chocolate bar. Maybe my son had just handed it to me. It was still early in the challenge and I remember him wanting me back on the sugar train.

I took that candy bar and held it. My hands were shaking and I started crying. Every edge from the previous three days was coming up and I realized that this was decision time. This was when I was going to step one way or the other and the voices inside of my head, the old Lizard Brain, all the habits, they all came forward with all their strength. It was the moment of truth.

I asked my wife to help me and hold me down. We had a massage table and she helped me lay down on it. My whole body started shaking. My arms couldn't stay still. My legs were twitching—classic withdrawals and detox.

It was the moment when I chose which side of the fence I was going to stand on for the rest of the 30 days.

It was never as hard after that day. And whether you've had that day or not, know that on the other side of it is a new strength that you'll remember for the rest of your life. What your Hero's Journey will look like will probably be different than mine, but it will show up.

Exactly how much sugar was I eating to prompt this level of reaction when it was removed for just 4 days? It wasn't obscene. Besides all the hidden sugar that was in just about everything I ate, I was good for a few desserts each week and a daily Snickers or Reese's treat. I would never say no to ice cream and once I discovered gluten-free cookies, I was an easy date. Clearly it was enough, however, that my body wasn't going to let go without taking me for one last memorable and scary thrill ride.

Day 4 is as memorable as my wedding day or the day my son was born. On hindsight, it was as equally defining as either of those two events.

The reason I put it into such a sacred category of days is because, as you read above, I just about lost it. Everything I knew and trusted was being tested.

I knew that if I got through that day, nothing would ever be the same, and I would be the superhero of my own life.

Face my demons and speak my truth in tough situations? Absolutely!

Hold people accountable and expect to be held accountable by others? Don't mind if I do.

Co-create a world-wide community of people who want to experience 30 Days Sugar Free and put myself out as a leader? No turning back!

What I found out about slaying the sugar beast is that it was really only the first step in opening doors of possibility in my life. And I'm nothing special. I've seen this happen for others who have walked past the temptations, squashed the naysayers, and stood strong in the darkest moments of this challenge.

Ground Zero for a Better Life

There's a lot of research supporting that inner voice that I've talked about. You know, the one that tells you that sugar is a poison and the less of it you eat, the better off you'll be.

The vision of what you want might be crystal clear while the steps to attainment are often murky and inconvenient. For thousands of years human beings have feared and resisted change. We are hard-wired to keep on keeping on—even if that means doing something we know is unhealthy, unsafe, or unintelligent. The familiar is comfortable. Change is not.

Fear of change can be paralyzing. Consider this cycle:

- Flash of inspiration about a change you can make in your life
- Surge of energy about how it will change your life
- Fired up – ready to act, create, develop, etc.
- One step forward, two steps back
- Convincing yourself it wasn't that good an idea
- Guilt about still doing something you know isn't healthy, safe, or intelligent
- Back to step 1

Have you ever found yourself dancing to this song? Somewhere deep in the Lizard Brain, we get the message that if we want to stay safe, we'd better not change. In most cases the fear of change stops us from taking any action at all. It calls for, and receives, support from its allies including anxiety, self-doubt, peer pressure, and the aforementioned guilt.

Don't worry—this isn't unique to you. It's typical, expected, and fixable.

It takes an ordeal of sorts to move past the status quo. This is the journey discussed in the chapter, *The Hero's Journey of Sugar Free*. If you take that journey and come out on top, the good news is this: you will never be the helpless victim when you want to make any change in your life.

What Does This Have to do With Quitting Sugar for 30 Days?

In *The Hero's Journey of Sugar Free*, I proposed that getting through a month without sugar was ground zero for a better life—inside and out. Sugar is the subject for the journey that I decided to write about because it attacks the fear of change on six different levels: mental, emotional, physical, physiological, chemical, and spiritual.

While you could take this journey with just about any life change that will shake up your complacency (exercise, writing, reading, organizing, finances, relationships, etc.), sugar offers a minute-by-minute reminder that will keep you present and in tune with the journey, the growth, and the transformation.

Sugar's effects on the human body are so destructive, and it is so immersed in our culture, that going off it for 30-days makes this the true Hero's Journey.

We all come out of the Hero's Journey with an understanding about our physical and emotional capacity that we never knew existed. We become superheroes in the realm of our potential.

Wishing you the strength to choose exactly what you want and need from this experience.

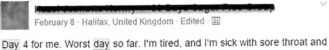

February 8 · Halifax, United Kingdom · Edited · 🔟

Day 4 for me. Worst day so far. I'm tired, and I'm sick with sore throat and aching body. As a comfort & mood eater, I'm missing my fruit cordial and comfort foods-cookies and the odd glass of rosé.
Hoping I feel better asap as its not helping my focus on 30 days sf 😔

But I'm sticking with it!!

Like · Comment · 👍 10 💬 9

DAY 5

Celebration and Slip-Ups

Y ou are one-sixth of the way through—the first really respectable fraction on the road to 30 Days Sugar Free.

While that is a very mathematical and analytical way of looking at it, the truth is that every single time you lift your hand to your mouth and make a choice to not eat sugar, you have done something very respectable.

Understanding that this is a very personal journey, I am sending you a huge literary high-five and hug of congratulations. Spend a few minutes this morning taking in the achievement of what you've done. I wish I was sitting there so you could tell me how it's feeling. Close your eyes and see yourself with a cape and a smile (or your version of your inner super hero). This will give positive reinforcement for the challenge. It is nothing short of spectacular.

Share the Achievement!

One way to open the circle of celebration is to let others know about your success. In the Member Area there is a link to download your very own Day 5 achievement badge. There is a new badge every five days! http://ILoveMeMoreThanSugar.com

Ideas on How to Use Your Badge
- Post the badge on social media sites such as your Facebook wall or Instagram account. You'll be entertained by the comments and

congratulations that come your way from people you might not have heard from in quite some time!

- Email it to a friend or family member.
- Print it out and put it on your refrigerator.
- Make a copy for work and hang it at your desk.

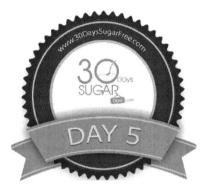

From the Glory of Celebration, Let's Land Back in Day 5

I want to talk to you about slips. Specifically, I want to talk to you about the available paths you can take if you have one.

September 23 ·

Note to self: It is not a good idea to help your friend, the organic chocolatier, pack boxes for the Fall pick up when you are on Day 12 Sugar Free, and not tell the friend you are sugar free.

No longer sugar free. I didn't gorge, but sugar passed my lips

Like · Comment · 💬 12

I promised right up front that there is nothing in this challenge that's about shame and guilt—and you can take that to the bank. There is enough of that available elsewhere in the world. I am going to cover the two ways slips can happen and a few ways to frame each so that you can continue on your challenge with your spirit (and dignity) intact.

Sugar On Purpose

That's right! Proud, bold, and unapologetically you walk up to that cupboard and say your version of, "Forget Barry and this silly challenge.

I deserve this cookie and no one is going to stop me! And while I'm at it—I'll have three."

Hey, it happens. My job as a coach for this challenge is to expose all the stories that otherwise live in the dark, private, shadowy places of the mind. For it is here, out in the open, that they are exposed and lose all their power to drive us towards behaviors that the bigger parts of us don't want.

So that happens—sugar was consumed. The raid is over and the pride and entitlement with which you attacked the pantry has subsided. You might not be sure exactly what to feel but the nagging voice of the 30 Days Sugar Free challenge may be part of your soundtrack.

You have two choices at this point and the path you take is completely up to you:

1. Go on like nothing happened
2. Tell on yourself—be accountable and still achieve the 30 Days Sugar Free

How Both of These Options Play Out—Immediate and Long Term

1. Go on Like Nothing Happened.
   This choice seems easy. You brush your teeth and you are back on the train. You carry a sense of courage forward that you learned your lesson and it won't happen again. And this might be the case. Historically, and for a few good reasons, it usually doesn't play out that way. You have broken an agreement and given some of your power back to the sugar habit. The parts where the habit lives are chalking one up in the "Win" column and they go back into the challenge a wee bit stronger.

2. Tell on Yourself.
   This choice seems scary. You finish the sugar and sit for a moment. You feel for any effects you notice. Increased heartbeat, grit on your teeth, tightness of muscles, or maybe even a different attitude or mood than you had before the sugar. You see, this is an amazing opportunity! In this moment you have a lot of data and power to use in showing the sugar habit that you aren't joking around—and

you are even going to take it a step further. You are to going check in with one of your sugar free supporters! By doing this you grab your sword and take a slice at the part of yourself that wants to keep sugar a secret. You also evoke support from someone who has your back! And while the sugar habit did get a taste of what it wanted, this could hardly be considered a "Win".

Sugar By Accident

You're at a picnic enjoying conversation with friends and there is a big bowl of coleslaw on the serving table. You spoon a hill of it onto your plate. You see baked beans and a hot dog with ketchup and you say, "Yes, please!"

We don't need to pick apart this train wreck—pretty much everything on your plate has sugar and you munched it down without thinking you were doing anything wrong.

If fact, with all the other sugary choices on the table at that picnic, you're thinking you did a pretty good job! It wasn't until maybe you felt a bit queasy, or a friend mentioned the recipe for the coleslaw, that you realized what happened.

Slips happen. I don't know your age but if you take your current age, it's pretty safe to assume that is how many years you've been eating sugar. The important gift that comes from a slip-up is that it gives you an added awareness to look at everything you eat during these 30 days.

Depending on how far you are into your 30 Days Sugar Free challenge, what you ate will awaken different dormant feelings and reactions in the body.

You have a couple of choices on how to move forward. Again, completely up to you:

1. Beat yourself up, call yourself names, and compare your intelligence to celebrities and politicians you dislike.
2. Show yourself to someone and move forward!

Choice #1 is just plain crazy talk.

Choice #2 is awesome. While you might be upset with yourself, it's a perfect opportunity to practice taking the lesson and ditching the shame. Walk over it. Keep your day count going and don't dwell on the slip up. Convert any guilt you have into power and focus moving forward. Reach out to someone you trust who has your back! The point in doing that is to be accountable to yourself and keep it from turning into a "secret" that empowers the sugar habit.

Now... Let's Get Back to Celebrating!

Engagement

Don't forget to use your Day 5 badge in a way that will inspire yourself and others. You'll get so many comments that will help you to keep going. It's harnessing the love of your network to support you in something that many of them might consider doing once they see you rocking the status quo! Others might just write, "You're crazy!" and that's fun, too.

Tomorrow we are going to get into the connection between the body and the mind when doing 30 Days Sugar Free. We might as well start with a bit of dancing right now! Can you put on a song and get up and dance? Do a personal victory strut for five days sugar free?

What does it feel like to move around with a system that has been sugar free for five days? Identify one feeling and put it in your journal. "Today when I danced I felt _____".

See you on Day 6!

DAY 6

Pushing the (Flesh) Envelope

Here's a letter that came from a very early Facebook group that I was a part of. I got permission to share it and a blessing from the author that she hopes it helps "even one person!" My guess is that it will do more than that.

It's official. Today is one year without sugar. This is a big deal. Not many people understand my addiction with this substance. It started when I was in my early teens. I was alone and would go up to the cupboard and just pour myself a glass of sugar.

It could be regular sugar, powdered sugar, brown sugar. Chocolate was my next level up. Just add cocoa powder to the powder of sugar. Mix a little milk in and I was high.

My addiction was not bad until my mid 20s and early 30s when I was diagnosed with Crohn's disease. My body cannot process real food. Now, my love affair with sugar and processed food flourished. It was the only food my body didn't reject. Add to the mix 16 years of steroids.

Yup, you guessed it. The many years of high doses of Prednisone made me diabetic. What is a girl to do? Keep eating the sugar and kill myself slowly or try to eat healthy and be very sick every day of my life? Of course,

I chose the sugar. I got off the steroids, diabetes went away. Unfortunately my addiction with sugar was there. I continued down this path for several more years. I woke up one day and decided to join Jenny Craig. This was the first good choice I had made in many years. I lost my weight, 53 pounds, but I never addressed my addiction. So as you can guess, it all came back.

Last August, two things happened. I started back on Jenny Craig again and started the 30 Days Sugar Free challenge.

The cravings are gone but my brain still says, 'Feed me sugar,' when I am stressed. So today I take out my Yonana Machine, make healthy ice cream, and celebrate a job well done. Gone is sugar from my life and I'm feeling great. —**Caren M., California**

Experiences like that encourage me to continue sharing the ideas of 30 Days Sugar Free with others. Caren has been such a model of what's possible, and watching her transformation has been nothing less than, well, transformational.

There are a percentage of people who go sugar free for medical reasons. There are others that do it voluntarily to lose weight, feel better, and a host of other reasons. I've been fascinated with that distinction and can't help but wonder which group has an easier time.

It's such a personal journey—the chemistry makes it impossible to compare any two people. What I do know is that going 30 Days Sugar Free is life-changing. It's a teacher of the highest order whose lessons come in all shapes and sizes. It's the sum of all you've eaten in your life plus who you aspire to be from this day forward. It touches every aspect of your personal and inner-personal life on a daily basis, and in the wee hours of the night, it's you who are left to reconcile the moments.

Hang in there and record the highs, lows, and in-betweens. That journal will act as a beacon during this 30 Days Sugar Free, and for years to come. Access to a journal of feelings, thoughts, and a life clear of sugar will give you a valuable perspective of who you are.

Moving Your Body

I want to connect a few dots that are important, and if properly integrated into this challenge, will streamline the road to shedding weight, sleeping better, detoxing from sugar, lowering anxiety, and overall health improvement.

I've said a few times over the past week that change takes change. You've been doing hero's work on changing the way you relate to food. Now I am asking you to alter your day to include 30 minutes of exercise that you haven't ever tried before. Anything from walking to mountain biking to dog sledding (we have Alaskans in the tribe!).

While many of you are already doing a regular exercise routine, I am asking you to break it and try something different. You see, sugar is a routine, too. Always there and dependable. You have broken that routine and now we are going to stack the successes with another kind of change—one of the physical body.

How and where does it land for you when you read that? Do you have resentment? Ease? Resistance? Excitement?

I am reaching in and turning one of the screws in your brain that didn't know it was going to be a part of this 30 days. The body, of course, is a part of everything we do. However, there is a tendency to think of it as separate; like it is something that just carries around the really important parts of us: the brain, the mouth, the eyes, the sexual organs.

Have you ever heard the following quote? – "How you do anything is how you do everything." I don't know who first said that quote, but I have spent years looking for a place in my life where it isn't 100% true. When I get away from the excuses I can so easily create about being late, unorganized, hyperactive, too generous with my time, or even unlovable, I see that how I do anything is how I do everything.

This is the essence of routine. It's the reason we can eat sugar when we know it's counter-intuitive to us living a long and healthy life. We tell ourselves it's fine. That escape valve is what allows us to say that so many things "are fine" when they really aren't.

Regardless of busy days, "idiots at work," bad drivers, or scarfing a plate of food that has nothing to do with who we want to be—there are themes that define how we behave and interact with ourselves and others. And those themes are the operating system of our life.

How you do anything is how you do everything

So for the rest of this 30 Days Sugar Free, can you agree to change how you do something (to, in effect, change how you do everything)? Can you try a few different forms of exercise for 30 minutes each day? It's exciting to pitch this out and imagine all the ripples this small change will have on your life—and those that you would have never met if you kept doing the same routine.

This switch-a-roo and physical integration of the body/mind will put a charge into your 30 Days Sugar Free. Take the risk. You could refuse... but that's not why you're here.

Coaching

While some of you might know exactly what exercise or activity you are going to try (maybe you've just been waiting for a good excuse or invitation), others might be feeling the mental equivalent of vapor lock. If that's you, here are my Top Ten ideas for you to try for 30 minutes and experience something that isn't the same!

- Juggling – get 3 plastic grocery bags and search YouTube – "How to Juggle Plastic Bags"!
- Hiking
- Swimming
- Dancing
- Yoga or Simple Stretching
- Walk/Run Alternating
- Driving Range (Golfing)
- Gardening/Landscaping
- Tennis
- Reading on a Stationary Bike

Grab an easy one for today and increase the distance from your norm in the days ahead. Who's going to be the first non-golfer to go hit a bucket of balls?! Come on—there's magic outside of the comfort zone.

This connection between the body and the mind is powerful. Exercise will enhance creativity and make you smarter. It will give you the gift of clarity and the motivation to keep showing up as who you want to be in the world.

Journal

Write down exactly what movement are you willing to commit to adding to your life. It won't take away from you—guaranteed. This is something that will give back in ways you can't even imagine.

Track your exercise for the next two weeks—what you did, amount of time, and your reactions. I'll check back in with you on Day 22.

DAY 7

Looking at the Inner Game

Somehow, you're here. A week without processed or refined sugar is probably a badge you never imagined being able to pin to your shirt. My respect for you is brimming and believe it or not, it's not because you've steered clear of eating sugar. Don't get me wrong— great work there—however the bigger handshake or hug is coming because you are winning the inner game of this challenge.

October 8 ·

Last night I came dangerously close to eating frozen yogurt--and then Halloween candy. Although it was Day 7, it felt like my previous Day 4, complete with crying and all. Fortunately, I remembered how crappy I feel on sugar and stopped myself. Phew!

Like · Comment · 👍 10 💬 11

Let's talk about the importance of that inner game, how it plays into this challenge, and how it's the framework for anything that is ever going to manifest in your life.

At the risk of stating the obvious, the inner game takes place within your mind. It's played against such obstacles as fear, self-doubt, lapses in focus, limiting beliefs, or assumptions. Your inner game, whether you know it or not, has a lot to do with you being here today. You've felt it. Heard it. Fought with it. Aligned with it. Now let's learn a few tools to honor it.

First—Recalling Prompts from Day 2 – Answers from My Journal

Here are some of those prompts from my journal that I promised you:

1. The reason I am doing this 30 Days Sugar Free is to:
   - Challenge myself to something that I feel is impossible
   - Experience what it feels like to deprive myself of something I enjoy as I have no experience in doing such a thing
   - Model for my son that with a mindset of success, difficult challenges don't stand a chance

2. What I think I'll learn about myself is:
   - I can do this
   - I will feel better without processed or refined sugar in my diet
   - I will find this to be harder than quitting gluten/wheat
   - I will have a new level of clarity around work and conversations
   - My body will love this and I'll wish I had done it years ago
   - If this 30 Day Sugar Free challenge goes well, I will want to go for a year

3. What I'm afraid I'll learn about myself is:
   - That it's yet another thing I'll fail at completing
   - I'll crack because I've already quit gluten/wheat and one more thing will make me edgy and unbearable
   - I'll become a pain in the rear to my family
   - I won't be able to find a way to "reward" myself after a workout or long work day
   - I connect a lot of my worth to food and the only good foods have sugar
   - I'll hate myself for always looking at labels
   - I'll slip up and put myself into a tailspin of guilt and shame

4. The clear list of what I will put aside for 30 days is:
   - All foods that list any form of processed or refined sugar on the ingredients
   - Restaurant salad dressings besides oil/vinegar
   - Root beer (Ouch!)

- Obvious violations like Reese's Peanut Butter Cups and Snickers
- My beloved sunflower butter (until I find one without sugar—I won't forget you!)
- S'mores by the campfire

5. The sweets I will continue to eat over these 30 days are:
   - All fruits and drinks that have natural occurring sugar—including red wine, which usually has less naturally occurring sugar than white
   - I will use less than 1/4 cup of raw, organic honey over the 30 days—a drop here or there

6. This is what completing 30 Days Sugar Free means to me:
   - This is the latest challenge in a life that has been driven by challenge
   - Completing it will give me a sense of clarity that I've only imagined or read about
   - It will be another thing for my son to remember me for when I'm gone
   - I hope it will empower him to know that he can do anything he wants
   - It will certainly open doors of opportunity for me—every challenge seems to bring its own surprises
   - It also means that at some point in my life I'll be able to call upon this experience to give me the power to take the steps necessary to complete the next challenge
   - When I'm done challenging myself, I'm done living

7. The best part of that will be:
   - Another level of knowing myself. Expand my edges
   - Never having to wonder what it feels like to be free of sugar for a month
   - Surprising my son with my superhero like powers of saying no to frozen yogurt, Reese's Peanut Butter Cups, and root beer. I love to surprise that kid!

OK, You Busted Me

Instead of talking about the Inner Game, I thought I would just show you. Journaling is among the most powerful ways to program yourself for success. It's a quiet, personal time that you can use to review and drive your inner game.

Journal

If you didn't respond to these prompts in Day 2, please go do them right now. I feel your heart in this challenge and I imagine you sailing free and easy through Day 7!

DAY 8
What Do You Expect?

Here we are, deep in the challenge, and you might be dancing between elation and frustration as the days unfold. Know that you are right on target. If you are here you are doing this perfectly.

I asked you to notice any changes. It's around this time in the challenge that I hear people saying one of two things:

- I can't believe how my body is changing, or
- Why aren't I losing any weight?

What we are doing for this 30 days isn't all about sugar! There—I said it. This challenge is about creating a deeper understanding about what you put in your mouth. We are using sugar as the teaching tool because it's been heavily influencing your life as long as you've been alive.

I want to be clear that simply removing processed and refined sugar from your diet may or may not cause any movement on your bathroom scale. There are many variables including:

- How much extra weight you were carrying before the challenge
- How much processed/refined sugar you were eating before the challenge
- What you are eating in place of the snacks
- How many other "legal" sugars like fruit juice, pasta, crackers, or other carbohydrates you are eating
- How many empty calories you are eating now that are not rich in nutrients or good fats

You might find some sugar free crackers that you really like and sit down with a big plate of them and some low-fat cheese and boom— you've had a higher calorie intake than if you slugged down a Snickers Bar.

It's a balance and that's why I say this challenge isn't only about sugar. You have given yourself this gift of 30 days to walk an exploratory route through your dietary landscape. After 7 days, I have heard from people who have lost between zero and 15 lbs. I've said it before and I'll repeat it here on this day, tame your addiction to processed and refined sugars and any other challenge you take on will be simple in comparison. There isn't a system of the human experience unaffected by the amount of sugar our culture eats. Develop maturity around that relationship and any other change you wish for yourself will look simple.

Expectations

These are really something, aren't they? Our expectations can determine how we feel—good or bad, happy or sad, angry or content, over what happens to us in a day, a year, or a life. They have an impact on how we feel about our self-image, relationships, job, and even people we meet at a party.

Are expectations met, or are they not met?

A lot of power can be handed over to expectations—and the truth is, rarely are they carefully planned out. Many times expectations are based on "best case scenarios" without a lot of room for Murphy's Law, reality, or even the occasional bad day.

If a company published their business projections the way people develop expectations, it would be impossible to attract investors. Expectations have no place in the driver's seat of our emotions unless we have put in the due diligence of planning. And this winds us back to our 30 Days Sugar Free journey, of course.

My goal in this challenge is to get you through 30 days without eating processed or refined sugar. That is the expectation. I have no expectation that you will reduce weight, become more agile, have more energy, lose your facial wrinkles, or lower your stress level.

Those are bigger goals that require planning. And while it's quite possible that any or all of those changes could happen to you during this 30 days, it's shaky ground to hold those changes as expectations. Are you getting the importance of what I'm saying here?

The one expectation you set for yourself can be measured and met very simply. You want to go 30 Days Sugar Free. I have discovered what it takes to support people through that challenge and my expectation is that I will successfully provide that support.

Adding to the List of Expectations

What if you want some or all of those changes mentioned above during these 30 days?

Good! I was hoping you would. How that happens is by planning, defining, and executing—just like the aforementioned business does when they create their annual projections.

· Decide on the goal
· Find what you must do to achieve it
· State a realistic expectation

Does that sound familiar? It's exactly what we've done with 30 Days Sugar Free!

Let's take one of those expectations listed above, run through the steps, and determine if we can set it as a realistic goal.

S.M.A.R.T. Goals

Expectations are met by achieving goals that are relevant to the outcome. For this, we will use the acronym S.M.A.R.T.

Specific – Is it clear, without ambiguity?
Measurable – Is there a number in it?
Achievable – Is there an action-oriented verb, for example, lose, complete, or weigh?
Relevant – Is the goal consistent with your expectations?
Time-Bound – Is there a deadline or expiration date?

S.M.A.R.T. Goals | Lose 5 lbs. During My 30 Days Sugar Free

Decide on the goal. Then run it through the steps: Lose 5 lbs. over the 30 days. That's a SMART goal.

Find out what you must do to achieve the goal: Removing all processed and refined sugar can definitely lead to this result. It's a great start. What could ruin the result is if you overeat a bunch of other foods that turn into sugar during digestion such as white flours, certain starches, fruits, etc.

State a realistic expectation: I will lose 5 lbs. during the next 30 days by stopping all processed and refined sugars and limiting my intake of foods that turn into sugars during digestion.

Now that is an expectation you can take to the bank! I'd invest in that one, no problem.

Taking This Out Into Life

I've told you that this sugar free experience is really a sneaky plot for you to be empowered to make any change you want to see in your life. This simple plan for developing expectations that you can meet is powerful and sets you up to win—time after time.

The takeaway is to constantly check in with yourself with these words: are my expectations realistic? Did they come from a S.M.A.R.T goal? If they are, then execute your 3-step plan.

· Decide on the goal
· Find what you must do to achieve it
· State a realistic expectation

If the expectation isn't met, it's a wonderful learning moment and one that I hope you won't waste with anger, abuse, depression, or fear. Instead, practice setting a new expectation and get back on the horse.

Earlier in the book, I mentioned my experience with the Tough Mudder race. It was my first time ever attempting something so outlandish and physically demanding. To recap, it involved a 10-mile run and 26 British Military Obstacles including 10,000 volts of electricity, barbed wire, wall climbing, and freezing water. My expectations were to finish the race—even if I skipped or fell off some of the obstacles—and come home alive. Success! S.M.A.R.T.

I did it again the following year and upped my expectations. This time I set the goal of succeeding on all 26 obstacles and coming home alive. I upped the expectation, so I stepped up my training. You can't raise your expectations without raising your preparation and commitment. *Quick report—I DID IT! Solid on all 26 obstacles including the inverted-V monkey bars—Woot Woot!*

With regard to the 30 Days Sugar Free challenge, get clear on your expectations, and be ready to meet them. Do all three steps and get real clear on what the second step must look like. Over-estimate, if you want to be sure.

Journal

Respond to these prompts in your journal:

- My expectations for the first 8 days were...
- My expectations for the next 22 days are...
- Extra "training" I will do to meet my expectations include...

I can't wait to see you tomorrow!

DAY 9
Dining Outside the Box

Final day of single digit days sugar free! Take a moment and breathe that in. It's a huge step for a human being in the 21st century especially because, as anyone will tell you, sugar is everywhere! You might be, for this one instant, the proverbial one in a million. You certainly are in my book.

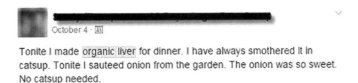

October 4 · 🔼

Tonite I made organic liver for dinner. I have always smothered it in catsup. Tonite I sauteed onion from the garden. The onion was so sweet. No catsup needed.

Like · Comment · 👍 6 💬 11

Let me guess—at this point you are nearing edges that you never knew existed inside yourself and pushing your comfort zone almost hourly. Thank you, and for my next trick...

Yes, you are deep in the reprogramming stage and it's not unusual to have flashes of what your life was like two weeks ago. "I could never do that" in regards to 30 Days Sugar Free is probably a joke to you now. That, if I'm guessing correctly, was a touchy edge for you before you started—way outside the comfort zone. Again, I want to say how honored I am to be a part of this experience with you. It's Day 9, and although you have probably faced this by now, I want to go deeper into how to handle the restaurant experience. Here I'll share more of my favorite survival tips for pulling off the sugar free experience outside of your own kitchen.

Dessert

Huh?—yeah, you know me by now, I like to shake things up so let's start at the end. You're full from a great meal (more on that below!) and now everyone is falling into the habit that has been well-established in our society—eat more! Put a big load of sugar on top of that food you just ate and *then* you're done.

What is the smart choice for dessert? For this 30 Days Sugar Free, the best choice is to check in with your stomach and see if you are actually called to eat more food. Dessert at a restaurant is rarely about satisfying a physical hunger. Be open to the message you get from your body, not the habitual or entitled voices in the brain. This month we aren't letting those voices rule the day.

After that check-in, you'll know if you are going to make a move toward dessert. If you are, go for a small bowl of fresh fruit. Watch out if it's fruit cocktail from a can. The syrup it's stored in is often a sugary blend that we are avoiding this month. If the restaurant doesn't have fresh fruit, try a mint or other herbal tea. Here on Day 9, your taste buds will give you some latitude—and your digestive system will thank you.

The Internet is Your Friend

Most restaurants will have their menu online and you can be prepared before you arrive. Your consciousness around eating over the past week is your ally as you sit down and they hand you the menu. If you are meeting a friend or family member at a restaurant and you have determined that the sugar free options won't cut it, there is nothing wrong with showing up 1/2 full and ordering a nice salad or appetizer as your main course.

Be Specific with Your Order

Right down to the bone! You are aware of the hidden sugars that show up in sauces, marinades, salad dressings, garnishes—don't be shy about describing exactly what you want. After a long shift (weeks, months, years!) of taking the same old orders, I've found that waiters are eager to satisfy a specific order and even become your teammate in making your experience excellent.

Remember—you might eat less. Be prepared to enjoy the company, conversation, and the foods they serve that fit your preferences. Restaurants are an easy place to slip. The more prepared you are before you arrive, the easier it will be to have a sugar free experience.

A Solid Rule of Thumb

Eat whole foods without sauces. Order a chicken breast, fish, or other meat and hold the BBQ sauce, salad dressings, ketchup, and au jus. Use oil/vinegar, lemon wedge, or Tabasco sauce to add a sugar free topping.

Parting shot on restaurants—I've never been shut out for going sugar free. I've been able to get by on every menu I've found and you can, too. Know that this is for 30 days and all those restaurant options will be there for you if you want them later.

Engagement

I'm going to recommend watching a stand-up routine by the comedian, Louis CK. This one comes with a warning—Louis CK swears. He uses profanity. It's meant for adult ears only and even then... the language in this clip might be offensive to some.

I also believe that his message is important to hear. It reflects a lot of the accepted attitude around food in our culture. His no-nonsense approach shines a light on something that often lives in the shadow places with other habits.

Again, and in bold this time, **this video contains profanity, swearing, bad words—and, the message is valuable.**

You can find the link to the video in the Member Area. http://ILoveMeMoreThanSugar.com

> *"The meal isn't over when I'm full! The meal is over when I hate myself!" —**Louis CK***

For this 30 Days Sugar Free—know that you're worth every bit of energy you're putting into this challenge.

A Day for Integration – And Another Badge!

Welcome to a banner day in your challenge. Ten successful days of consciousness around what you put in your mouth places you in an elite subcategory of the general population. Without any scientific data to back it up, I'm imagining similar-sized groups might include lottery winners, people who have been in outer space, and those that can fall asleep to bagpipe music.

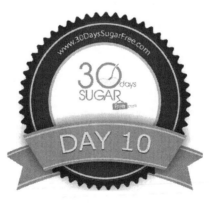

You've broken into the double digits and that is news worth sharing. In the Member Area, you'll find the link to download your Day 10 badge. Share this monster of an accomplishment, will you? When I see these, they always put a huge smile on my face!

The benefits of sharing your challenge may reflect back to you a hundred fold. It only takes a minute and you have no idea who in the world it will inspire to take a look at their own relationship with food and sugar. Download your badge from the Member Area for Day 10. http://ILoveMeMoreThanSugar.com

Where Are We on Day 10?

What a ride we have been on so far. In groups and in emails from those who have gone before, I've seen courage, compassion, self-examination, and varying forms of the "Big Why" for doing this challenge. What a gift for me to be on the witnessing end of all that truth.

We dug into the snack pantry and separated out a handful of quick go-to snacks. Make sure at least one of these is with you at all times. Often the difference between a success and a slip is a small bag of almonds/raisins away.

We looked at the archetypal story of the Hero's Journey through the lens of 30 Days Sugar Free. We discussed slipping off the program and dipped our toes into the pool of guilt or shame and found that, all told, we are better served by using our experiences to strengthen our character and commitment.

On Day 6, we added something to the mix that will integrate our mind and body so our entire being is working the challenge. On that day we also contemplated that *how you do anything is how you do everything*. That expression might have landed pretty deeply—in relation to this challenge and more of life. Not surprising.

You took a deep glance inside my head with my responses to the "Big Why" prompts, and hopefully you dug deep and wrote many of your own reasons for doing this. I'm sure in ten days you've already wondered, more than once, why exactly you are on this path at all. Normal. Expected. Stay here.

We examined expectations and looked at them through the eyes of S.M.A.R.T. Goals. Of course you can, and should, apply this to any area of your life including relationships, education, and health. I just have a soft spot for running everything through the lens of 30 Days Sugar Free for this challenge.

We looked at dining out and how to keep your eye on the goal when someone else is doing the cooking. I think back to my Day 10 and remember that restaurants (and, of course, airport food courts!) presented some of the shakiest ground during those early days.

Journal

Spend 15 minutes with your journal. Here are a few prompts to get you going. Feel free to use your own if you have other ideas that are more important or personal to you.

- I have noticed a greater awareness around... (moods, feelings, my abilities, etc.)
- I have noticed these changes in my relationship to food (desire, quantity, frequency, taste, etc.)
- Something I'd like to tell myself when I am feeling weak in this challenge...

Engagement

Where are your urges compared to where they were two weeks ago? Are you more able to walk easily by bowls of candy, random acts of sugar, or even your old favorites? Do you feel less temptation to eat sugar? Does today feel less like you're white-knuckling it and more like you own it?

Remember that person I asked you to find who really wants to see you win? I'd like you to check in with them and read them the responses to the prompts above. It will be good for both of you.

Celebration Food

Here are the ingredients necessary for making your own power bars. These are sweet, delicious, and your sugar-eating-friends will take one bite and accuse you of cheating.

Simple list of ingredients:

- 8 ounces of raisins
- 1 bar unsweetened 100% cacao (baking section)
- 1 cup of almonds

See the full recipe along with photos in the Resources for Day 10 in the Member Area for Day 10. http://ILoveMeMoreThanSugar.com

Trust and Intelligence

When you bought this book and started the challenge, you put some level of trust in me. Without knowing me, you invited me to have some input into your daily life.

By documenting my own journey and talking with hundreds of others attempting sugar free challenges, I created what you are holding in your hands. There is no Sugar Free University where I could get a diploma in teaching or coaching you in something so specific. All of this took a lot of trust—on both our parts. We each had to go outside of our comfort zones to open this relationship. You could have looked away when you saw the book—but those lips on the cover were hard to ignore, weren't they? I could have had the idea for this challenge and then let it slip away. We've all let ideas slip away, hundreds of times. So where did that trust come from? Why are we in this 30 day challenge together?

I have a theory. At the moment of decision, we each followed our Gut Intelligence. On this singular occasion. we each put aside the logical voices in our head and allowed the prehistoric part of us to take control and say, "This is what must happen right now."

Hawaiians call it the Na'au—or Gut Intelligence

I mentioned the na'au, or Gut Intelligence, in *Your Big Why*. I remember when I first saw my dear friend, Tony Bonnici, wearing this shirt—*live in the na'au*. We were at a workshop and he gave a short presentation

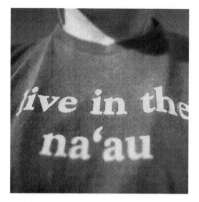

on the na'au and how listening to it always led to the answer that was right for you. We had three days together and he invited each person at the workshop to trust their Gut Intelligence at least once each day. Well, that challenge has never quite let go of me and I share this photo with you along with the same invitation.

Shared Attributes of the Gut and Brain

Many hormones and chemicals previously thought to exist only in the gut are indeed active in the brain. These include: insulin, cholecystokinin, vasoactive intestinal protein, motilin, gastrin, somato-statin, thyroptropin releasing hormone, neurostensin, secretin, substance P, glucagon, and bombesin.

And if that doesn't connect enough dots of relationship between the brain and the belly, consider this: both move through 90-minute cycles in the sleep state. The brain in your head does slow-wave sleep frequencies, immediately followed by rapid eye movement (REM)— that's when you dream. The lower stomach's cycle consists of slow-wave muscular contractions followed by brief spurts of rapid muscular movements.

Insert theme from The Twilight Zone!

But what voting power are you granting a gut layered in fat? If you are feeling shame, sadness, guilt, or anger about your gut, are you likely to give it a voice in making decisions?

We are in the thick of this challenge and for the next 20 days I want you to pay special attention to the knots in your stomach, belly aches before a challenge or test, butterflies in your stomach, diarrhea when you're scared, or that gut instinct. Allow that intelligence to win the debate and embrace the outcome.

You're here—right now. This is the time to step over the carcasses of old stories and deputize that gut of yours—regardless of your past relationship with it—and to grab the reins as you ride toward the transformation you desire. As questions come up for you about whether this or that ingredient is allowed as part of the 30 Days Sugar Free, or whether you should or shouldn't eat some particular food, I ask you to touch into your Gut Intelligence—your na'au—for the answer.

My umbrella comment over all of these questions is this: can you eat for 30 Days Sugar Free in a way that isn't questionable? Can you treat yourself to the experience in such a way that you're sure what you are eating is whole food free of any processed or refined sugars? After the 30 days, your taste buds will be so different that you'll be in a position to really choose who you want to be in relation to all the food options.

Journal

Respond to these prompts today. I ask you to be vulnerable and open as you go deeper than you ever have with yourself. Tap into the Gut Intelligence for your responses.

- When in your life did you feel something in your gut but let the logical brain in your head talk you out of it?
- What was good about the outcome?
- What *might* have been different if you followed your gut?
- What will you commit to resolve by following your Gut Intelligence?

Be on the lookout for the messages from below. They hold your truth. What a relief it is to lie down at night knowing that you followed your gut wisdom.

Great work! I'm so happy you're here.

DAY 12

Where Sugar Hides

Here on Day 12 you are pretty much an expert on what you are eating. If you are getting ready to try something new, check both the Nutrition Facts label and the Ingredients. If you see sugars listed in the Nutrition Facts, cross check it with the Ingredients to see where it's coming from.

October 6 · 🗓

Hey folks, here's a reminder to always read the ingredients, no matter how "healthy" the packaging looks! My one encounter with sugar during the program was because a friend told me he cooked the chicken in salsa. Since salsa is generally sugar free I had a small portion. Immediately I got my IBS symptoms back and had to go to the bathroom. When I came out, I asked him what kind of salsa. "Newman's Own!" he said. "That's healthy stuff, right?" We fished the bottle out of the trash and checked the ingredients. Sure enough, sugar was one of the ingredients. I was new and inexperienced. Now I know. But be very careful of processed "healthy" food. Even from Newman's Own.

Unlike · Comment · 👍 4

Let's look at some other places that sugar hides.

Medicines

I was checking labels for some of the most popular drops and syrups and wasn't really that surprised to find that many contain sugar (under one of its clever names). Sugar might make these syrups and drops taste better, but does it make any sense to have something in a medicine that your body is going to have to fight off? Since your system is busy enough just fighting off the cold, flu, infection, or fever, don't give it extra work to do. Healthy foods, including soups, broths, and extra liquids, will do wonders for improving your health.

I am not advising you to discontinue any medicine. I'm not a doctor, clearly. I am doing as I always do—helping you to be aware of sugar and how it might show up in places you haven't imagined.

Condiments

Ketchup might just be the ultimate mating of sweet and savory. People have become very creative with delivery devices to get ketchup into their body. The obvious: French fries, onion rings, and potatoes. Then there are the artists among us who have used ketchup to adorn eggs, grilled cheese sandwiches, and even pizza.

The truth about most ketchup brands is this: tomato concentrate and high fructose corn syrup. Hunt for alternative condiments that are healthy including salsa, Tabasco sauce, or oil/vinegar dressing. I was the champion of ketchup consumption back in the day. Hold tight—the craving does go away and you're better off for it.

Meat

In its natural form, meats are all free of added sugar. Where it starts to go wrong is when processing, sauces, or seasonings come into the game. It's possible to find bacon (think Pederson's brand) or hot dogs (Hebrew National) without added sugar. Check the ingredients and be armed with the 50+ Names for Sugar list.

These are small infractions and the ones that I really want you to watch for the first 30 days. The awareness is one aspect of this challenge, along with the health benefits of steering clear of sugar completely.

Journal

What has happened so far with this challenge that isn't sitting quite right with you?

- Have you talked about it with someone you wish you hadn't?
- Did you judge anyone else as "better" or "worse" because of a reaction they had about your 30 Days Sugar Free?

- Is there a belief you have about yourself that you haven't voiced since you started?

Those are three topics I expanded upon in my journal around Day 12. That writing helped me to really understand more about the role sugar has played in so many parts of my life.

Do some writing and examination on that prompt: what has happened so far with this challenge that isn't sitting quite right with you?

What comes from this day of journaling can humanize what you are feeling inside that might feel shameful, dark, or even wrong. You are messing with your DNA over these 30 Days Sugar Free and the more connected you are to yourself, the more centered you'll be through the transition.

To succeed in this challenge, you've already used more than brute willpower. Keep peeling back the stories so that you can touch the truth. That stuff is an antidote to the Lizard Brain.

Engagement

Do your body two additional favors which won't take an extra minute of your time! How's that for a win/win?

At this stage of the challenge, your body is in a full-blown detoxification. Make no mistake, there are negotiations being made between different cells in your body that have never even met. Borrowing fat, lending glucose, and even sharing workloads. Right now your body is trying to figure out if this is the new way of being or if you are going to cave in and return to business as usual.

So in support of the former choice, first and foremost—drink more water than you have ever imagined possible. Keep the inside of your body lubricated and flushing. Don't make it work any harder than it has to during this period of detox. If you feel thirsty, you waited too long to drink. Second, find a deeper level of satisfaction in your breathing.

If you can, and I hope you can, pick three times during your day to simply close your eyes and take 10 deep breaths.

Use this pattern:
- Breathe in slowly through your nose—fill your entire belly first and then chest for a full 5 count.
- Hold that breath for a full 5 count.
- Exhale through your mouth, slowly releasing that breath for a full 10 count.

Breathe deeply, laugh, and I'll see you on Day 13.

Breaking Bad – Habits and You

I have done a lot of study around habits. It's been one of my missions to learn about them and how they control human behavior, limit us from reaching our goals, and scare us back into playing it safe. Recall from *Living in the Habit* that there are two kinds of habits—Unconscious and Conscious.

Where Are You Focusing?

How I wish I could tell you to "just stop it" and you would! Heck, I wish I could tell myself that. But habits don't work that way.

The most effective way to break or develop a habit is by carefully choosing the focal point. "I don't want to bite my nails" is a great goal, but the subconscious holds onto pictures, feelings, and actions. That good intention of yours won't bring you any closer to a brilliant set of fingernails because the brain hears and stores the picture and action of what you've been doing (because that's what it knows) and the action it can extract from the sentence is: "I bite my nails." Not exactly the message you are trying to send home.

"I won't eat sugar" equals "I eat sugar" and guess what? Chomp. Chomp. Yeah, that's right.

Here is a technique that is as simple and powerful as drinking a glass of water first thing in the morning (and I want you to do that, too).

We are going to dwell in the realm of pictures and feelings, so let's go!

5 Steps to Re-writing a Habit

Get really clear on the habit you want to break. I mean, get down to the micro detail level. Pretend you wanted to teach me how to do your habit. What are the cues, steps, and feelings that I'll recognize? How will I know when it starts? Ends? This is really important for this process and I want you to take a few moments to write out the exact habit you are going to let go of today.

Take everything that the habit is to you: feelings, judgments, emotions, reactions, history, costs, and anything else that comes to mind. Write it onto a piece of paper with as much detail as possible. Hold the piece of paper once you're finished and read it over. Did you miss anything? Are you holding back or selling yourself short? Don't!

Now put this aside and get a new piece of paper. On this one we are going to focus on the feelings and images of you after this habit is removed from your life. In at least as much detail (hopefully more), outline your life, sleep, health, relationships, body, energy, and anything else that will be improved once this habit has been eliminated. You can write, draw, or mix it up. The goal is to create something that motivates you and makes you feel successful. Feelings and images speak to those parts of your brain.

This step requires a tad of choreography but if you're able to walk and talk (simultaneously), you got this covered. You are going to destroy the first sheet. Tear, shred, burn, crumble, beat with a tennis racket—whatever it takes for you to emotionally and physically release all that is held by the current habit. Do this safely without causing harm to yourself, others, or any property.

And now, because nature's way is to instantly fill an empty space, you are going to read aloud everything from that second page while looking at it. Connect your subconscious mind with what getting rid of the habit is going to look and feel like. From our example above it would go like this: "My fingernails are beautiful and… " that is when you begin reading/seeing what life is like on the other side of the transformation. Your new association to fingernails is everything on that 2nd sheet of paper as you manifest it into your life.

Focus—where we put it equals what we get done in life. Speak to yourself in terms of already having the desired outcome and it will be your focus, which, with trust and commitment, will be your new habit.

5 Steps to Re-writing a Habit: Cheat Sheet
- Dissect the habit you want to break.
- On a piece of paper, write what it means to you.
- On a second piece of paper, write the benefits you'll experience when the habit is gone.
- Destroy the first piece of paper.
- Read aloud the second piece of paper.

This is your time to master the inner game of habits. This simple technique works so well and can be applied to anything from exercise to studying. You didn't get the habit overnight and it will take some time and commitment to change it. Do this as needed and stay strong.

Coaching

What is another habitual behavior you have that you would like to re-define?

Here are some possible categories and there are dozens more:
- Financial responsibility
- Piles of paper or clutter in your home
- Other eating habits
- Exercise routines
- Time management
- Communication
- Relationship skills

What small step can you take today or begin after the 30 Days Sugar Free? Imagine applying what you have done with the sugar challenge to create another conscious habit?

I encourage you to take this momentum and roll it into the next place in your life that would benefit from a behavioral overhaul.

After you do two or three of these in a row, the skill of being able to re-write habits will become the habit and you won't even have to think about the steps.

This is the arena of giants. And if you have some story about yourself not being a giant—stay tuned.

On Day 17, we are going to rewrite those stories and put that one to rest.

Engagement

Define your next 30 day challenge and decide when you are going to start. Keep it specific, just like this challenge. Note a few thoughts and actions that are helping you succeed with sugar, and know that you can take those with you into the next challenge.

Adapt *5 Steps to Re-writing a Habit* to apply to another aspect of your life.

Spend time on this. Use your journal and write the bestseller that is your new relationship to food. With that chapter in place, your life is going to become a lot more vibrant and enjoyable.

DAY 14
What Are You Noticing?

Welcome back and I really want to say, "You Look Mahvelous!" Who are you now with two weeks sugar free in your permanent record? Remember in school when they threatened you with putting something in your "permanent record"? Does anyone even know where that is? Well, if you find it, add the fact that you have completed two weeks sugar free! That, unlike a lot of the historical details in there, is newsworthy.

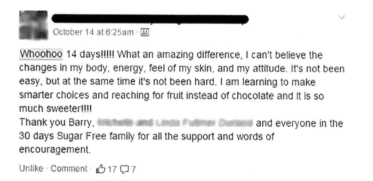

October 14 at 6:25am ·

Whoohoo 14 days!!!!! What an amazing difference, I can't believe the changes in my body, energy, feel of my skin, and my attitude. It's not been easy, but at the same time it's not been hard. I am learning to make smarter choices and reaching for fruit instead of chocolate and it is so much sweeter!!!!

Thank you Barry, ████████ and Linda ██████ ███████ and everyone in the 30 days Sugar Free family for all the support and words of encouragement.

Unlike · Comment · 👍 17 💬 7

A special note if you've had a slip in the last two weeks: You are here with us! The slips that happened were realized and explored. I imagine you've seen a side of yourself and sharpened your sword. Those conversations or journal entries where you showed yourself—vulnerable and open—sent a powerful message to various parts of your psyche. Those moments are as much a part of this journey as the sugar free moments.

Today is a day to build some momentum for the final push of this challenge, and wouldn't you know it? I have ideas to help you do exactly that.

There are Two Groups of People at this Point in the Challenge

First Group – To those of you that are feeling extremely comfortable and confident about riding this challenge home with a burst of energy, hooray! Huge props to you for doing the work, following the coaching, and shutting up the parts of the ancient brain that fear and resist change. You are leaders and no doubt inspiring those in your immediate circle and around the world with your courage. You may or may not be getting this feedback—or even willing to let it in. Please do. It's a service to those around you if you let their comments land and be acknowledged.

Second Group – I also know that others of you are wondering why you are doing this and if you should keep going. You aren't noticing any weight loss or big physical changes. You're tired of waiting and feeling like you should be seeing some results by now.

Remember those big slow breaths from Day 12? Let's take one together right now. There... already feeling better, right?

What Changes Are You Noticing?

If you are in the second group, I am going to zoom out the lens for a moment so we can gain some valuable perspective. Give me some latitude here to dig under the scab, if you will.

First off, we're not talking about numbers on a scale or size of pants. Everybody is different.

I can tell you that it is impossible to be at this point in the challenge and not see and/or feel some changes in your body. What is probably more accurate is that what you are seeing and feeling isn't meeting your hopes and expectations.

For a moment, forget about what you think you *should be* noticing at this point in the challenge. Let's talk about what you *are* noticing.

Go down to the micro level, because this can be very subtle:

- sleep pattern/quality
- digestion or elimination
- skin tone/texture/appearance
- mental capacity or clarity
- energy levels throughout the day
- your mood cycles
- any of the senses, particularly olfactory (smell) and taste
- less junk food wrappers on the floor of your car
- dozens of other possibilities!

You didn't become who you are overnight and you aren't going to undo it overnight, either. It is of paramount importance that you take the time to notice and record the most subtle changes you have seen in yourself, your environment, or your relationships in the past two weeks. Remember how the Lizard Brain hates change? Those tiny indicators might be all that your brain is allowing you right now in hopes that you'll get over all this nonsense and come back to what it knows and loves—the version of you that you chose to leave behind two weeks ago!

Coaching

Let's go in for a closer look. I'm going to be blunt here—what are you doing, and what are you not doing, from what I have suggested over the past 13 days? If I were there with you right now and looking you in your eyes, what percentage of the coaching could you tell me that you have followed?

Granted—it has been a lot of content over the past 13 days. I know that and I front-loaded it on purpose. It has been the long-distance version of picking you up and shaking you. Quitting sugar demands that kind of rough handling because of its addictive properties and secret handshakes it has with certain parts of your brain.

It would be very hard for anyone to do all of what I have prescribed. My question to you is this: did you select the parts that were easiest for you, or did you reach way outside of your comfort zone and try the ones that scared the heck out of you? Did you tell yourself that some of the coaching ideas "don't apply to me because I am different/

already knew that/have tried it before/don't believe in that" or any of a hundred excuses that were safer and easier than doing it?

Come on... I've been watching people do this for awhile now and you know it's true. I got your number on at least a few of these places you've let slide.

Engagement

Do you know what? You're going to finish this challenge with me! Could you take a few minutes right now and go back over the past 13 days. Check the Coaching or Engagement sections and be open to one of the suggestions you blew off for one of the reasons mentioned above—or maybe one I didn't mention. Make sure it's a suggestion that when you first read it you told yourself you weren't going to do it—but this time do it!

Which coaching suggestions will produce results you'll see and feel? All of them, of course, or I wouldn't have mentioned them in the first place. Here are a few of the simplest that you might have shied away from at first reading:

- Eat a high protein breakfast.
- Drink water at least every fifteen minutes while you are awake—keep a refillable bottle handy.
- Journal! If you are expecting to track your progress just in your head, you'll never recognize the changes. A lot of your brain isn't in favor of this change and it'll mess with your memory and results.
- Exercise – did you add something NEW to your routine? I suggested 12 options that easily fit the bill. Same old will yield you the same old.
- Try the breathing system highlighted in Day 12.

Those are just a few of the coaching/engagement ideas; the low hanging fruit, if you will. Truthfully, everything in this book is here to offer you a variety of ways to sneak up on the habit-brain. If the only bit of my coaching you are following is not eating sugar and you are mad that your pants aren't yet loose, we need to talk!

Let's make this experience spectacular. What you want is yours for the taking. Don't let it slip away.

DAY 15
Completing the Past

Happy Half Way to 30 Days Sugar Free! Is it just me or did that two weeks fly by in the blink of an eye? Seems like we just started this challenge and bam—halfway home!

The good news is this: experts agree that at this point the chemical addiction is all but over. After two weeks of no processed or refined sugar, your body isn't demanding it like it was in the early days. If you are still feeling pulls toward sugar, just know that it's a lot less than it was and you are making huge progress. Right now you are working mostly with habit, social pressures, convenience, and that good 'ol entitlement. We have worked with ideas and techniques to address all of that. So what's left?

The 3 P's of the Next Two Weeks: Practice. Presence. Persistence.

Of course, this challenge could crumble like a house of cards and your Lizard Brain would be more than happy to pick up where it left off. How about this: stay the course for two more weeks so you can experience how it feels to have your body free and clear of processed and refined sugar for 30 days. From personal experience and all reports I've collected—it's glorious.

Practice – As you well know by this point in the challenge, this is a practice. You get better at recognizing and refusing sugary foods. You've increased your ability to refocus your attention onto what you are creating, instead of what has always been. Stay with the practice.

Presence – Slips happen as fast as the lift of a hand and a swallow. A big part of this challenge is being present in places where we used to be loose and sloppy. Put a toll booth on the bridge that has always had free passage between hand and mouth. Make sure you are aware of what exactly is requesting permission to board.

Persistence – Have you been around a kid that just keeps asking and pushing for dessert? They are creative geniuses that come up with deals and reasons faster than a defense lawyer. There's a lot to learn from them. Over the next two weeks, I ask that you channel their persistence and turn it on its head. Make the deals and reasoning work for you to stay sugar free. You've got a belt full of tools to help you at this point.

Share the Love

In the Member Area you'll find the link to your Day 15 badge.
http://ILoveMeMoreThanSugar.com

Seeing that you are 1/2 way through this challenge will probably encourage a few people in your life to:
·   Examine their own relationship with sugar
·   Know they have a trusted support partner in you if they want to do it
·   Congratulate the heck out of you for making it!

Journal

What are you absolutely loving about this challenge?

While it's usually easier to express what we aren't happy about, the positive reinforcement of consciously speaking about what you really love is far more productive. I'm not going to get all *The Secret* on you here. (You know that movie? Very mystical!) Just suffice it to say that if you share something you love, chances are those around you will do the same.

If you are complaining about life and what's going on—you'll get more of that in return.

Journal for 15 minutes on all of the positives of this experience.

The Completion Process

In 2010, I was a student in a coaching program called Human Potential 2.0. It was run by a man named Bill Lamond who was a founding member of the personal coaching profession. He is a remarkable leader that taught me a lot about trusting my voice in the world and clarifying how I want to show up. He speaks internationally for corporate clients and I feel blessed to have had those 10-weeks with him.

In the program I did with him, Bill spoke about the Five Pillars of Freedom. A year later I was checking in with him about how those pillars have been playing into my life. I told Bill that I used what he calls his Completion Process to completely stop a habitual compulsion that had haunted me for over 35 years. I then had the honor of interviewing him about his Pillars of Freedom. He gave me permission to share the recordings with anyone who could benefit from them—and that is certainly you!

The Completion Process is a fast and simple way to take all of the random data you have about a subject, relationship, incident, or belief and put it into one single folder—and delete it. This remarkable technology is only one of the five powerful interviews I share with you in the Member Area.

Outline of a Completion

You'll hear the entire explanation in the interview. In addition, I want to give you a template that you can use to run the Completion Process as often as you like.

State the current belief about the topic or relationship to the person/topic:
1. What's good about it?
2. What's bad about it?
3. Who do I need to thank for it?
4. Who do I need to apologize to?
5. What else do I need to say to be complete?

As you'll find out in the interview, you can do this Completion Process with any behavior, addiction, attitude, or experience to help move yourself into a different state.

In the Member Area for Day 15, you'll find links to each interview. They are short and concise. Please listen to them in order as they build on each other. http://ILoveMeMoreThanSugar.com

There are a number of completions you'll want to do around food and sugar as this is a hot topic here on your two-week anniversary. Those are covered in the second interview. In the third interview, Bill shares the Installation Process where you get to define your future belief or relationship with a person, topic, or behavior. Listen to these in order. They are short, so please don't skip ahead.

Engagement

If you haven't already, this is an excellent time to share with a friend what you are doing. You are lit up and glowing—unlike many of the sugar-filled zombies that are walking the earth. This glow of yours might just sway someone who's on the fence to give it a try, too. Sometimes it only takes a ray of light to help a friend see what they've been looking for.

Go listen to the interviews and do a few Completions & Installations today. This technology works on a very deep level while you are busy doing other things. Brilliant.

DAY 16

What's at Risk?

L et's get right into something that might be happening below the surface of your 30 Days Sugar Free challenge.

Are you living with someone that isn't doing this challenge? If you are, there is the reality that here on Day 16 it might be presenting challenges, tension, judgments, or even anger with your family or housemates.

This challenge of yours brings with it an energetic shift in the dynamics of a household. It touches everything and everyone who lives there. It happens in some ways that are overtly obvious and others that a video camera would never catch.

The glaring differences are easy: more fresh foods, less wrappers/ boxes, new labels and logos in the cabinet/refrigerator, and radically different snacking habits—just to name a few.

The concealed changes might include others feeling like they are "less than," "better than," guilty for eating their foods in front of you, self-conscious about their choices, or even resentful of you and your commitment.

Both of these lists could go on and on, limited only by the dimensions of the human personality.

The real question is, why would any of this ever happen? Why can't we all just get along?

How many people have said something to you about this challenge and you got the feeling that what they said to you wasn't really about you? In the chapter, *Living in the Habit*, I touched on how your doing this challenge is a mirror to those in your life: family, co-workers, friends, and even someone at a party that sees you skipping the dessert table.

Has someone said something about you in the last few weeks that, on hindsight, wasn't really about you at all?

After my first week sugar free, a friend at the gym said, "Your skin has changed so much in the past week since you quit eating sugar!"

That sounds like it might be about me, right? Well, here's the context that I left out. We were both in front of a mirror and he was staring at his own face. In particular, a big, shiny zit that had just surfaced was under military-style investigation. And while my skin might have looked better, what really served this man was the change he saw in me and how it related to him. It's our nature.

> *"We don't see things as they are, we see them as we are."*
> —*Anais Nin*

We are Mirrors for Each Other

During interactions with others, while "people watching," at the movies, and yes—even right in our own home—humans have this remarkable ability to see in others what they want, have, or lack in themselves. Dozens of comparisons happen every minute while we seamlessly carry on with our conversations or engagements. I want you to be aware of these comparisons that happen right in your own home. There is nothing unnatural about this. It is as it has always been.

While it is interesting to watch and interact with other people, the brain is primarily using the input (visual, auditory, and olfactory) to reconcile common ground.

When you see someone you like that is funny, sweet, personable—it is a safe bet that those qualities reside in you. When you see someone that you consider loud, obnoxious, rude—you are probably seeing parts of yourself that you dislike or have disowned.

My son has a very sweet friend, Teddy, who is bright-eyed and wears his emotions, open and unguarded, right on his face. I asked him how school was going and if there were any kids that got on his nerves.

"Yes," he said, "a kid named Ellis."

"Oh," I said, "what does Ellis show you that you don't like about yourself?"

I watched his face go from confused, to smiling, to curious. "He's really rude sometimes", Teddy said. Then he added, "I guess I am, too." I love that kid. Not a drop of pretense anywhere on him!

While you contemplate all of that, let's bring it around to our 30 Days Sugar Free.

What's at Risk?

Is there a living soul that believes they should be eating sugar? I'm not talking about wanting, or deserving, or enjoying—I mean is there anyone that believes it really helps them in terms of health, longevity, or physical conditioning?

Of course, sugar is expected and accepted in our culture, but I'm talking about the truth that lives deep in you. Are there people who believe that added sugar actually helps them be who they want to be? Live the life they want to live? That eating 150 lbs of sugar every year supports any of the goals they set or dreams they have? Probably not.

Drop that dark little truth into a home with someone that is doing 30 Days Sugar Free, recall the fact that we are all mirrors for each other, and there is a test tube where interactions can get hot and heavy. Bear in mind, the dissonance will take place under the surface and will manifest itself in more mundane talking points such as clothes on the floor, dirty dishes, or leaving the lights on. A deep, meaningful heart-to-heart conversation might reveal what's really going on.

The risk that someone would have to take to come clean might sound something like this: "Your actions threaten me. I can't see myself ever getting through a single day sugar free and you are over two weeks! Everything in me envies you for doing this and a big part of me wants you to fail so I can see you as I always have."

Coaching

What can you do to ease any tensions? You can understand what's going on and be aware of the story that is playing out. Be sensitive to others that are walking the party line on food and drink. In addition to everything else they have going on in their life, they are living with a mirror that is providing them a front-row-center view of a part of them that they might not want to see.

> *"Be kind, for everyone you meet is fighting a battle you know nothing about."* —**Wendy Mass, The Candymakers**

Remain a clear example of who you are. Shy away from mentioning the sugar free lifestyle at all—they know about it and dealing with it is really their work. You're doing yours.

If they ask you about your sugar free challenge, be vulnerable and honest. Share the struggles and triumphs. That transparency is a welcome mat for them to share what they are really feeling/experiencing. I've seen it dozens of times and it's pure magic.

Engagement

Go to the Member Area and watch this inspirational video on the Day 16 links: *TED Talk, Matt Cutts: Try Something New for 30 Days*. He spent a year doing something quite extraordinary which is inspirational by any measure. His story is especially poignant during this challenge. What were the people close to him seeing reflected when they watched him? http://ILoveMeMoreThanSugar.com

Matt's spirit epitomizes what you are doing with this challenge. You'll get a special chuckle at 2:53!

At this point in the challenge, I see people start to take more ownership and responsibility for what they say about their choices. The honeymoon is over and now it's personal. With that shift might come new levels of sensitivity around comments from others. Whether it comes in the form of a joke, advice, an I-told-you-so, or even a confession, know that none of it is about you. You are walking a new edge in life that is new to you and everyone you know. Keep your hand on the rail, your eyes in front of you, and your focus on the work.

The moments where you feel yourself closest to an edge are the moments that are most meaningful. Today's successfully navigated edge is tomorrow's comfort zone. This expansion leads to an increased capacity to be your bigger self. Keep dancing on the edges!

Parting words for Day 16? This challenge is looking really good on you. Shine on you crazy diamond!

The Stories We Tell Ourselves

Welcome back. Your commitment to show up and do the work, day after day, is inspirational. What you are doing for yourself and your circle of influence is life-affirming. It's a vote you cast in each moment to honor yourself and the people you love. Hold that as a guiding light as you navigate Day 17 and make sure to take it into your heart. You're doing this because you care about yourself.

Now that you are firmly into the double-digit-days of sugar free living, are you finding more of a pattern and less panic? Exit surveys from my online program point to a wonderful statistic: in anywhere from 7–10 days from now, many people will be free from the habit of eating processed or refined sugar.

This is YOU we're talking about! Not someone from *People Magazine* or a story featured on *60 Minutes*.

You have created this for yourself and honestly, it's a miracle in today's sugar-filled-and-frosted world.

Huge props to you—and now let's keep doing the work.

What Stories Are You Telling Yourself?

What if you had a superpower that allowed you to listen to the stories you tell yourself about your life: abilities, limitations, talents, compassion, love, creativity, or control, and know instantly if they were true or not?

Let's face it—there are a number of people that live in your head—from boisterous inner-critic to meek people-pleaser—and not all of them paid to get in! They each have a voice that comes in from time-to-time to "help" you and prevent your getting hurt. They can be insulting, rude, embarrassing, or even conceited.

Picture this—you are about to go to a party and you hear the voice in your head that says, "You don't look good in that dress," and a buzzer goes off. You are assured that the voice was false and you go to the party and have the time of your life—receiving over a dozen compliments on your dress.

Now, imagine you are at dinner on a sixth date with someone and you hear a voice in your head screaming, "This is the one! This is the one!" Instead of instantly clogging your brain with cross-examination and doubt, your superpower gives you the confidence to pick up your napkin, wipe your lips, look across the table and say, "I love you. What are you doing for the next 50 years?"

In lieu of this superpower, I am going to share with you a few ideas about the stories we tell ourselves, how we can reclaim the power they steal from us, and a way to mute them—dead in their tracks.

Where Do The Stories Come From?

We may not know where the stories come from. They are typically an amalgamation of many influences including childhood wounds, bad experiences, a negative presence in your immediate circle (past or current), and excessive exposure to media (news, television, political streams, magazines that say we could be better if we would only _____), and many other possibilities.

The Cost of Negative Stories

At best, these stories are bothersome. At worst, they paralyze. Many people find a place between those poles where they can function, prosper, but probably fall short of what they'd consider thriving. The stories usually pop up at key moments when decisions need to be made—at forks in the road when you have to choose between taking a risk with big rewards or taking the well-worn path back to safety.

Coaching

It's time to reclaim your power from the negative stories. You have already stepped over a big carcass of a story by making it to Day 17 in your 30 Days Sugar Free challenge. I know the voices that have taken a swipe at you over the past couple weeks as you ramped up and then began this challenge.

You have already done what it takes to reclaim your power from negative stories so you know, without a doubt, that the power to do it lives within you. You've done it many more times in your life, too. For illustration purposes, I am pointing to this challenge as a very recent victory over the chorus of negative stories.

What are two or three deliberate actions you took that enabled you to accept the 30 Days Sugar Free challenge?

Did you:
- Reach out to a friend/partner for support?
- Put your money where your mouth is?
- Make a deal with yourself that you'd just "try it" and quit if it wasn't working?
- Whip past the voices and make the decision from a place of conscious power?
- What else? Dig deep here and write down what you did to overcome the story.

Journal

List the stories that almost kept you from doing this challenge such as:
- This isn't the right time
- Barry's not the right coach for me
- It won't work
- I'll try it later
- … or any others.

Now list some tools you used to overcome the stories:
- Trusting yourself
- Confiding in a friend
- Listening to a higher power
- Putting one foot in front of the other
- Focusing only on the present moment
- Picturing the celebration at the end
- Bragging rights

- Heeding external motivation from others (kids, doctors, friends)
- You've always loved a good challenge
- A nagging curiosity that got a hold of you

Engagement

This is such a personal path—which is why I just had you write a list of your own tools for stopping stories before they get a hold on you.

Now it's time write your own prescription. Develop a one/two punch to stop any negative story the second it begins. Refer to your above list of tools and pick your two most powerful allies to combat a negative story. This is brain reprogramming and I want to promise you one thing: whether or not you believe it will work, you're right. Choose wisely.

Notice a negative story starting to play out in your head.

Take one deep breath/hold/release. Don't concern yourself with the story. Do the breathing.

Implement your one/two punch (two tools) from your journal and let them overpower the story.

Repeat steps 2 and 3 as needed and picture a door closing on the negative story.

Make this a practice and it will become second nature. Soon, you'll need to do it less and less each day.

When will you practice it? You have a chance every single time a negative story starts playing in your head—in bed, in the shower, waiting in line, or even exercising. Don't wait for everything to be perfect!

Keep blessing yourself with more of this kind of care and respect. Rewriting your story is poetry.

Standing in the Fire

I get so fired up about meeting you here each day. I hope you can feel it even though time and space separate us.

I've received feedback from readers who tell me that the material in these pages is supporting them in the challenge AND in the rest of their lives. That's certainly what I see as the bigger possibility—and getting off sugar for a month isn't a bad by-product, right?

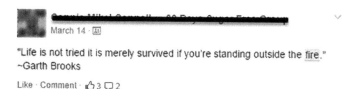

March 14 · 🔒

"Life is not tried it is merely survived if you're standing outside the fire."
~Garth Brooks

Like · Comment · 👍 3 💬 2

Let's talk about something that you have been demonstrating so well over the past 18 days. It's what gives you the power to say no to sugar, and why it gets easier every time you do it.

Standing in the Fire... This phrase comes up a lot when I'm talking to coaching clients. What does it mean to stand strong in the face of change, challenge, conflict, or confrontation? What is the conversation you have with yourself when faced with temptation? What does it do to you—during and after—to stand strong and look into the eyes of the opponent (even if it's a donut)? What does it mean for you to slink away or not show up because you are afraid of losing?

In the case of the 30 Days Sugar Free, we have opportunities to stand in the fire every day. At parties, restaurants, social gatherings, and right in our own home, opportunity presents itself! Some of us that live or work with other people are forced to see foods we are choosing not to eat. We have constant exposure to foods that have added sugar and have to develop a thick skin so that we are not in debate every time we walk through the kitchen or into the break room. And this is an excellent practice for the bigger game outside of the sugar arena.

My Secret Agenda

I want to give you encouragement to come up with at least one new area of your life where you can stand in the fire.

As a parent, a boss, employee, friend, entrepreneur, artist, or partner—there are opportunities to stand in the fire at every turn. Each time you choose to be in the presence of conflict, you can use what you are doing with this challenge to empower yourself to see the other side with compassion and understanding, yet still stick to what you know you need. Every time you make this choice you come out with more confidence. That confidence will make subsequent challenges much easier.

For instance, would you miss a party because someone you don't like will be there? That is certainly one way to handle it. What message, however, does that send to the visionary in you? Is this the way you want to show up or is it simply more comfortable? Getting clear on that distinction will give you valuable information about how to move past it, if that is what you want to do.

Here at Day 18, I would trust you to show up at a dessert bar and enjoy the presentation, company, and atmosphere. Seriously, if you were going to grab a slice of cheesecake you would have done it by now. Is there somewhere in your life that you are standing in the back, with one hand on the exit door, when the real healing and growth happens up a little closer to the stage?

Coaching

Get yourself a nickname for the person you are in this challenge. You don't have to share it with anyone unless you feel that will benefit you. It could be an animal totem name, a superhero name, or a character you invent. Make that fictional version of yourself the person that stands in the fire during your tough moments of this challenge and anywhere else in life.

Mine? Since you asked, it's Truthful Rhino! I picture my sturdy body, pointy horn, fearless posture, and I stand in what's harder to do because I want it more than I want to run.

Here are few others I've heard:
· Sugar Free Goddess
· Cowgirl Ninja
· Determined
· No More Ms. Puffy
· Wonder Girl
· (No)SugarMan

While doing your breathing exercise from Day 12, close your eyes and visualize this version of yourself. Hear the nickname in your mind a few times while you are exhaling. This action will speak to your subconscious. It's such a fun exercise and from this day forward you will have a name to call out to evoke that part of you that is courageous, compassionate, and centered enough to stand in the fire.

Engagement

Here is a follow-up from yesterday where I shared a 4-step system for getting the negative voices out of your head. It works—perfectly—and it will take some practice and trusting. It's for you and it has to be done by you. Stand in the fire and run these 4 steps on a story that's holding you back.

Negative Story 4-step Review:
· Notice the negative story.
· Take a deep breath/hold/release.
· Use your one/two punch (two tools) to overpower the story.
· Repeat as needed and picture a door closing on the story.

For another approach at quieting the negative voices and stories in your head, I want to share an entirely different solution.

Since laughter is great medicine, let's follow that path and heed the advice of the one, the only, Doctor Switzer. Go to the Member Area and watch the video for Day 18. http://ILoveMeMoreThanSugar.com

Here are some lyrics from a powerful song by Garth Brooks called *Standing Outside the Fire*. These lyrics are spot on brilliant for what we are doing here. We have to listen to ourselves and those advocating on behalf of who we can be in this life. The naysayers and pessimists don't deserve a vote on our life choices—this 30 days or beyond.

Until the very end, know that I'm standing in the fire of this challenge with you.

Outside the Fire

"But you've got to be tough when consumed by desire
'Cause it's not enough just to stand outside the fire
Life is not tried, it is merely survived
If you're standing outside the fire."
—Outside the Fire, Garth Brooks

Food and Time

Does it seem like the last 19 days have gone fast or slow for you? It's an interesting contemplation—how does our diet play a role in our perception of time. Does a 3PM crash make the day seem longer? Do the times when you stand in the fire of a sugar craving and walk away have an effect on the passage of time?

These are all good insights that I hope you'll add to that book you're writing to yourself.

Fun with Food

There are some very creative sugar free recipes in cookbooks and on the Internet. Note that most will use some alternative sweetener that we aren't using during this challenge, so get creative!

It's exciting to find a new recipe that I haven't cooked before. Substituting sugar (or alternative sweeteners) with pureed dates or eliminating it all together and adding more fruit or a few drops of raw organic honey—such a rewarding part of the challenge.

The longer you are sugar free, the more sensitive and discerning your taste buds become. I have gone from pouring honey onto apples to make them edible, to having to sit down and prepare for the intense sweetness of a plain Fuji apple!

Pretty radical change to take place in one lifetime. Shifts like that are expected and common during the 30 Days Sugar Free challenge.

What food or drink tastes different to you at this point? Share the answers in your journal or with a trusted friend. The reflections will anchor the positive changes in you more deeply, and that is valuable in giving you the strength you'll call upon in weak moments. Small wins add up to major victories.

An Important Research Paper

In my travels on the sugar free path, I met a remarkable young woman named Alex Curtis of SpoonfulOfSugarFree.com. She has a fantastic website and later in the book, I share an exclusive interview I did with her. She has also written a research paper that will help you understand the heroic job you have done of putting aside sugar over the past two-plus weeks.

In her paper, *The Psychology Behind Sugar Addictions*, she points to a study where lab mice were given access to limited amounts of sugar. They started wanting more and more. They were soon like little sugar-addicts. It's not hard to substitute "human" into her entire paper and see the exact treadmill we have been on for most of our lives—minus these last two weeks. Huge work you've done so far. Hats off to you!

Here is a summary of the main points of Alex's research paper:

We "Feel Better" When We Eat It. Eating sugar increases the serotonin levels in the body, which is a calming and mood elevating neurotransmitter. Serotonin plays an important part in regulating pain levels and sleep cycles, and it is an anti-depressant. When sugar levels increase, serotonin levels rise and individuals can feel better about themselves both physically and mentally.

It's as Addictive as Drugs Like Cocaine. Ingesting sugar can also increase dopamine levels, which is also what happens when someone ingests cocaine or other addictive drugs. This can cause a binge and withdrawal cycle and lead to a dependence on the substance.

The Brain Thinks it is Rewarding. The orbitofrontal cortex is an area in the front of the brain where humans process rewards, and this is activated when someone consumes sugar. Therefore, sugar is seen as rewarding to the body.

Engagement

Alex's research paper is well worth the time as it will give you more context for where you've been and where you're heading. I'm going to keep this page short so you can go read it. You'll find the link to her research paper in the Member Area for Day 19.
http://ILoveMeMoreThanSugar.com

Keep that smile on your face! Your eyes are brighter, skin is healthier, and although you might not actually feel it, the inner workings of your body are celebrating you.

DAY 20
Celebration Foods

Here you are—the 20 Days Sugar Free version of you is alive and more beautiful than ever! First Off—Check the Member Area for your Day 20 badge. http://ILoveMeMoreThanSugar.com

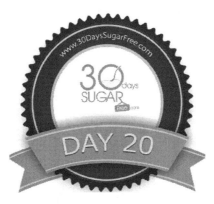

I said it before and it's worth repeating—you never know who you'll inspire to examine their relationship to sugar, all because they want to look, feel, and be like you!

I'd shower you with a full page of accolades and high-fives if I thought it would serve you. The truth is, you know what a rock star you are right now. In a very personal way you are the living embodiment of possibility and transformation. Your beauty shines.

Instead, let's use our short time together to do a quick review of the last 10 days and then keep the needle moving on our progress.

Where are We on Day 20?

I introduced you to something you've known your entire life. I asked you to hand over the fancy verbs and nouns of the analytical brain and trust your gut intelligence. This area of your body has an ancient knowledge of you and is standing by waiting for you to give it the nod to take control. Listen and trust it when you can't figure out an answer.

We examined a few of the less obvious places sugar rears its ugly head. At this point in the challenge you are a ninja label reader. Keep filling your knowledge base with the names of violators. You'll be a champion at the *Sugar: True or False* game in no time.

There were powerful journaling prompts that invited you to look at how this challenge is showing up in your relationships with others and with yourself. Hopefully you dove in and uncovered something that can help you in other areas of life, too. Remember, this challenge isn't really just about sugar! The breathing exercise on Day 12, for instance, will be a good friend to you for the rest of your days if you make it so.

An extensive look at the different types of habits and how to rewrite them came at the perfect time—including a five step system for rewriting them. Get in the practice of giving yourself permission to change, and the world will be your oyster.

I asked you to closely examine yourself for what you do notice in terms of change. I'm sure at this point you're getting comments from friends and family about your appearance. Even if the scale isn't changing all that much, weight tends to redistribute as puffiness deflates without sugar and the skin adjusts.

I shared the Completion Process and I hope you played with that. I remember the day I was introduced to that system by the creator, Bill Lamond. He walked me through it and in less than 5 minutes, I said goodbye to a haunting and troublesome mental glitch which had been with me since childhood. Step right up, my friend, and risk letting go of something that is no longer needed.

"We don't see things as they are, we see them as we are." Anais Nin offers this quote and it nicely sums up the experience others might be having around us during this challenge. I submitted that housemates will find their own way to deal with your sugar free diet. You are doing your work and that is where your focus needs to stay. Don't try fixing anyone!

All the world loves a story, but sometimes the stories we tell ourselves wreak havoc with our self-image and reality. In Day 17 I had you look at some strategies you've used thus far to reclaim your power from the stories in your head. It's your personal playbook for keeping your bright future in the cross hairs.

Standing in the Fire of change and refinement is another skill you've practiced plenty of times by Day 20. Your feet know well the feeling when your brain says "run," yet they refuse to budge. Transformation isn't for the meek, nor is Day 20. Shine on!

Finally we examined the way food plays into our perception of time. I've heard so many people say they can't believe how fast the 30 days goes! I have to agree.

I don't know when you're reading this, but I can tell you that November 25, 2014 marked Day 1,000 for me—and it really only seems like yesterday I was ripping open a Kit Kat bar. How are you feeling about time and food?

Journal

Let's keep some documentation going as it will always be there to show you who you are.

Set aside 15 minutes for these prompts about sugar:
- How are you talking about your 30 Days Sugar Free and how is it different than the way you spoke about it before you started?
- How have the stories you tell yourself about your relationship to sugar changed?
- How do you show up more confidently around not eating sugar?

And now, because I really like to show you how this is much bigger than sugar, jot some words in response to these prompts about your life:
- How are you talking about yourself and is it different than it was before you started?
- How have the stories you tell yourself about your relationship to challenges in life changed?
- How do you show up more confidently than you did before this started?

Engagement

Here are two of my favorite celebration foods/recipes for you to consider here on Day 20. You're two-thirds of the way through this challenge and I really think it's time to spice up the treat roster. With your taste buds continuing to return to their alive and sensitive state, let's toss two sensations your way that will reward the work of the last 20-days. One sweet, and one savory!

Kale Chips

The ultimate savory snack that is so good you could swear it's sweetened. This recipe comes from a 30 Days Sugar Free alumni who loves making these in her dehydrator (but can also be made in the oven).

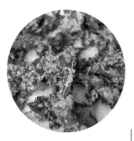

Kale Chip Recipe
Simple to make and watch out
—they go FAST!

1 bunch of organic kale
(I prefer curly kale)
2-3 Tbsp olive oil
1/2 tsp salt
1/2 tsp pepper
1 tsp garlic granules
1 tsp sun dried tomato
1/4 C nutritional yeast
2 Tbsp sesame seeds

Thoroughly wash the kale and cut into small, bite size pieces. Toss in a bowl with olive oil, salt, pepper, garlic granules, sesame seeds, and nutritional yeast. Work it around until all pieces are covered. Spread the pieces onto the dehydrator trays and run on medium for 4–5 hours.

These can also be made without a dehydrator using your oven. Preheat oven to 250 degrees. Spread the kale on a baking sheet in a single layer and bake for approximately 20 minutes (turn over the kale after 10 minutes). Make sure to keep them in until they are crispy and slightly browned but not burnt.

Chocolate Peanut Butter Celebration Cake

Alex Curtis, from SpoonfulOfSugarFree.com and the author of the research paper in Day 19, offers us this remarkable treat. All those good ingredients and a taste that just feels good going down. It's gluten, soy, dairy, grain, and sugar free—and tastier than you can imagine.

It's a great way to spoil yourself without breaking any of your 30 Days Sugar Free commitments.

See pictures and learn Alex's recipe by visiting the Member Area for Day 20. http://ILoveMeMoreThanSugar.com

DAY 21
Pattern Interrupts

Three weeks sugar free! Those words might stir up a myriad of emotions. Don't try to figure them out right now. The past can't be changed. The future hasn't happened. And in this moment you are consciously choosing to gift your body, mind, and soul by staying clear of processed and refined sugar. Period. That's all that's true right now.

You've no doubt been in a restaurant when a waiter drops a tray of plates. Conversations stop. Thoughts are lost into the ether. A joke being told might never get the laugh it deserves. This is an example of an accidental Pattern Interrupt. For the sake of this challenge, and your life moving forward, I want to talk to you about intentional Pattern Interrupts and how they can empower you to make better choices.

In Day 13, I discussed habits. I outlined a simple and powerful process for changing the focus from *words explaining what you don't want to be doing* to *the feelings and images of the desired behavior*. I hope you have put it to use for the last seven days.

I want to talk about another form of breaking habits. This one uses another part of the brain to distract us from the habit or behavior and put us instantly into a new reality.

A Pattern Interrupt is a conscious change of focus or physiology to stop a certain thought or situation from continuing down a known path. It's a simple-to-remember physical or vocal action that derails the pattern and is a valuable addition to your life's toolkit.

Habits are warm, fuzzy blankets to the Lizard Brain. They show up physically, emotionally, verbally, and socially. Their job is to keep us safe from change which, of course, is the Kryptonite to that part of us that wants things to stay just as they are.

Although I'm sure you could quickly form a list of your habits, here are a few examples from my life:

- Walking around when I'm on the phone
- Opening the refrigerator when I'm bored
- Interrupting my wife when she's going to tell me something I did that she didn't like
- Reading Facebook instead of doing what is on my daily agenda
- Talking first when I see my son instead of waiting for him to speak

What do all of these do to keep me safe from change? That's a discussion for another time, but I can clearly see these behaviors as habits or patterns. Repeatable, predictable, mostly unconscious, and dead center of my comfort zone. For all five of these I have Pattern Interrupts in place—and they work gloriously.

Word of the Day

Perturbation – a deviation of a system, moving object, or process from its regular or normal state of path, caused by an outside influence.
A two dollar word for Pattern Interrupt—at no extra charge!

Right now, I'm going to coach you through setting up a Pattern Interrupt that you can try today—right when you notice a pattern that you'd like to stop.

First Off – Identify a Habit

You knew I was going to ask you to do that, right? Identifying a habit is a bit like telling on yourself, however, you can do it right in the privacy of your own mind. I suggest writing the habit on a piece of paper so you have the experience of truly owning it as yours.

Next, to make this as simple as possible, I want you to look at the list below and grab the first one that sparks your interest. The further these are away from an action you would normally do, the better.

- Snap a rubber band that's on your wrist
- Sing the chorus from a favorite song as loud as you can

- Jump up and down 10 times and count the jumps in a foreign language
- Pet your dog
- Drum a rhythm onto a desk or counter
- Drink a glass of water
- Take a one minute power walk
- Splash water on your face
- Do five squats
- Slap your forehead three times quickly

Do you notice what all of these have in common? You can do them quickly, you don't need big props, and they require no thinking. Win. Win. Win.

Why Would You Want to Do This?

Let's be honest here. This little food challenge you have been living with has brought some foundational change to your life. It's impossible that you cut out all processed and refined sugar for more than three weeks and you are still experiencing life in the same way. That said, it's a golden opportunity for you to look at other habits or patterns in your life, the toll they take on you and others, and how they are holding you back from what lies ahead.

The place you're at right now—beating sugar's hold on you—is too valuable a position not to tinker with other patterns in your life. Pick one pattern, then pick an interrupt and run it for the day.

What Do I Do After the Interrupt?

After using a Pattern Interrupt, you do whatever you want except continue the pattern you were interrupting! Chances are that since you identified the pattern and did the interrupt, the urge to return to it isn't going to have a chance. If you do still feel the pull of the pattern, repeat the interrupt a few more times and even add in another one. These suckers are ancient and scared of your power. You can and will conquer any pattern using interrupts, the Completion Process (Day 15), and a deep commitment to change.

Tomorrow we'll take a step to seal the deal on your commitment.

One more week to go... all this looks really good on you!

A Look at Capacity

It's been a full day since we last met and talked about habits. I couldn't be more curious—what came up for you while reading that page?

Did you take a few moments to reflect on what you've done in the past three weeks and acknowledge yourself for taking on and tackling that Everest-sized habit? Here in the countdown days it is vitally important that you fill your memory bag with dozens of benefits, changes, compliments, insights, and takeaways. It's this momentum that will help you to create a healthy relationship with sugar—one that will serve you well for the rest of your life.

In what might seem like a lifetime ago—Day 6 to be exact—I challenged you to find something new to add to your exercise routine. I asked you to step up and find something new to do that moved your body in a way that would catch it off guard—sort of like you did 22 days ago when you took away its lollipop!

I gave you 10 ideas that you could do to confuse your body and get it out of the routine. Hopefully, you did at least one of those—maybe more? Did you, perhaps, combine a few of them and try juggling while dancing? In those early days it was important for you to keep throwing change at your brain.

What is Capacity?

I've mentioned the word "capacity" a few times over the past 21 days. What does it actually mean in the context I am using it?

Think of your refillable water bottle. Those come in sizes from the little 8 oz. model all the way up to the 1/2 gallon size. The size you have is probably perfect for your needs. Typically, by the time it gets low, you have a replacement jug or you are back in a place where you can re-fill that bottle. That bottle never changes size. It has the same capacity now as it did when you bought it.

You, on the other hand, have the ability to expand your capacity. With a few simple steps, you can accommodate your biggest dreams and scariest challenges.

On Day 15, I introduced you to the Completion Process. This is a world-class tool for expanding capacity. Combine that with the Installation Process and suddenly there are no limits. That's right— no limits. Your capacity to achieve, produce, or create expands to accommodate your willingness to face challenges. Over the past 21 days you have asked more of yourself and your capacity to deliver has stood by you.

Journal

Let's look at a variety of categories and journal about capacity. Write the word CAPACITY on the top of a new page and respond to these prompts. Rate your capacity on Day 22 vs. where it was when you began this challenge:

Category	Before Challenge	On Day 22
Conversations		
Overall Presence (focus)		
Willingness to Eat Healthy Foods		
Confidence		
Compassion		
Taste of Foods		
Senses (smell, hear, see, feel)		
Patience with Self and Others		
Physical health		
Emotional Balance		
Sleep		

Coaching

Are you willing to notch that up a few steps? I am asking for sweat, warrior cries, and maybe even an expletive or two aimed squarely at me. I can take it!

I challenge you to do an exercise routine that is ridiculously outside of your comfort zone. I'm asking you to raise your exercise capacity. And since I'm not there to tell you what to do, I am going to ask you— what would get you sweating, crying, and swearing (metaphorically, of course)?

In addition to the exercise options listed in Day 6, here is another list of possibilities. Aim for your comfort zone plus 25% where applicable:

· Biking
· Cross Training Class
· Spinning Class
· Jumping Jacks
· Weightlifting
· Rollerskating
· Paddleboarding
· Indoor Rock-climbing
· Hang-gliding
· Planking
· Zumba, Nia, Jazzercise, or other dance class
· Hoola-Hooping
· Join a Running Club
· Ultimate Frisbee
· Carry your child or grandchild
· Lovemaking

This is the day to do an extreme check-in with your body and see what you are capable of achieving. My guess is that your capacity has dramatically increased and you might not even know it—yet. Your hiatus from sugar has gifted you in so many ways—don't miss the opportunity to feel your new edges.

Engagement

Exercise—the act of moving your body—is what I want you to connect with here on Day 22. I'm not suggesting you do anything dangerous.

I simply ask that you push yourself further than you would if I didn't throw down this gauntlet.

From where I sit, it seems like you are ready to spend some of the juju you have built up over the past 22 days and I want you to reinvest it into your own body. Do this! Take this challenge from your coach and make yourself proud. Share the news with your friends if you want.

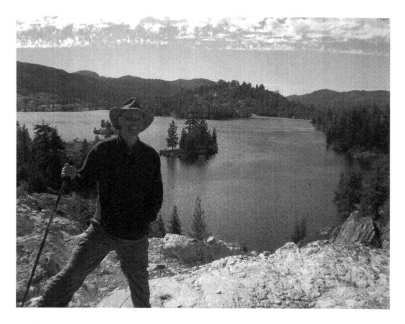

And just so you know I'm not sitting around cheering you on from a Lazy-Boy recliner, here is a photo of what I did last weekend with my sugar free self! I climbed to the top of a mountain overlooking a beautiful lake in the Sierra Mountains.

Have a great Day 22. You deserve it. Go out and live the only life you can—yours!

DAY 23
Lifestyle

Question: Is this feeling less like a white-knuckle roller coaster ride and more like your life? Day 23 is when you can toss around this simple-to-visualize sentence: "Only one more week to go with the challenge!"

Seriously—from here on out you are delivering daily blows to mortal remains of your sugar habit. You are fully detoxed, clear-headed, and have rebooted your taste buds. You would be shocked at what "sugar" tastes like if you decided to partake.

This journey began about three weeks ago when you turned the page and decided to give it a go. At that moment you were probably feeling one or more of these characteristics:

- Strength
- Insanity
- Desire
- Curiosity
- Skepticism
- Weakness
- Hope
- Or ???

Think back to that moment and picture where you were sitting. What you were wearing. What was the last sugary thing you had to eat and did that play into your choice to take on this challenge? What did you feel right after you decided? I am asking you to go back because whether or not you realize it, you are a very different person right now. Inside and out you are so far away from who you would be without that moment of decision and the brilliant way you've played it so far. Small moments of decision are the catalysts for huge change—and that person in the mirror is living proof.

Speaking of changes in the mirror—I really want to share this story about a very dear friend named Michele Rothstein with whom I do a lot of work in the world of sugar free living. She is my partner in our online program and such a positive, supportive coach for people around the world.

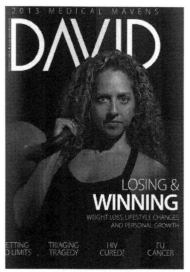

Michele looked into a mirror a few years ago and decided she wanted to see a whole new version of herself. She had a surgical jump start and from that day forward has been committed to her sugar free life. And look at that photo—would you mess with that determination?

A picture of Michele before she decided it was time for the next chapter of her life. I love her and her determination to never let the past dictate the future.

From Michele's Biography:

I struggled with my weight all my life. My parents sent me to 'fat camp' when I was in 6th grade. I went from 160 to 130. In 9th grade, I was on a strict protein shake diet for three months. I went from 190 to 160. All throughout high school I was well over 200 lbs.

I was always the 'funny girl'. The first one to poke fun at herself

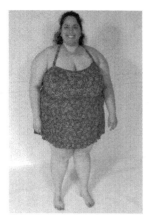

before someone else could. In college, I went on a doctor supervised program and went from 260 to 180. It didn't last long. I always went back to my old ways which included an endless amount of sugar.

By the time I decided to have gastric bypass surgery in 2005, my weight had reached an astonishing 359. One of my rules after surgery was NO SUGAR.

I couldn't imagine life without sugar, but I knew that my health was in serious jeopardy.

With a lot of hard work and dieting, I lost 200 pounds within the next year. But I still hadn't found it within myself to give up all processed and refined sugars. February 24, 2012 I decided it was time—I decided to give up sugar for 30 days. I felt so good that I decided to keep going. Why would I want to go back to the 'drug' that sends me on a downward spiral?

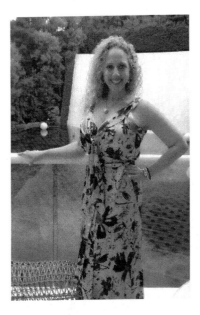

—Michele Rothstein, August 25, 2012

These days you are likely to find Michele doing yoga, running a marathon, or taking a trip around the world.

Coaching

Would you be willing to take a small risk right now? (Seems I am asking you to take a lot of risks, right?) Would you check in with someone close to you and ask them what changes they have noticed in you over the past few weeks? Get someone who has known you for a long time. It doesn't matter if they know about your sugar challenge or not.

Be open to whatever they say—and take it in without taking it personally. In other words, listen, register, and then don't make any drastic changes based on what you hear. Whether they have a laundry list to deliver or if they say, "What do you mean, changes?," just stretch yourself to be curious and vulnerable enough to ask for an outside reflection. It was on the 19th day of my challenge that my wife told me that for the first time in 25-years she had witnessed me IN conversations, instead of AT conversations. I've never forgotten that moment and it was a reflection that keeps me from ever wanting to go back.

Wishing I could see you right now!

DAY 24
A Letter to You

Let me turn up the music of reverence to honor you for the achievement of 24 days sugar free. And yes—I am including you even if you are thinking, "Well I did have those few 'slips'." Let that story go.

Take a slow, deep breath, put your hands on your heart, and take it in. You are here—conscious, present, and focused on another day of treating your body and soul to healthy eating and being. While that might seem ordinary to you at this point in the challenge, I offer the reflection that it is a rare and beautiful occurrence.

In the body of this daily page, I will guide you through the process of writing a letter to the future version of yourself.

I didn't do this when I started, and here I am, late in my sugar free life, wishing I had! How fantastic it would be to receive a letter from that scared man that sat on the couch shaking and crying on his Day 4.

This is something that I absolutely believe will serve you well a year from today. I'd like you to do this regardless of your plans for sugar after Day 30.

I'm including this in the book because I recently did mine! Of course, the best time would have been when I started my challenge in February of 2012, however the second best time is when I thought of it last week—and I grabbed it!

Logistics

You can do this either on pen and paper or an electronic device. I decided to go with pen/paper. I am writing my letter based on the prompts below, sealing it with the Open Date printed on the front, and hiding it somewhere safe.

In my calendar, I marked a date—one year from the day I wrote it—and put a reminder of where the letter is located—and that will be the day I open it!

If you want to go electronic, there is a free site that will email the information on a specific date and time. It's linked in the Member Area Resources for Day 24. http://ILoveMeMoreThanSugar.com

Prompts

The idea of this letter is to speak directly to yourself with the entirety of who you are today. Beyond the sugar challenge, speak from the parts of yourself that have fought the battles, overcome the temptations, and taken the Hero's Journey.

Write about who you are and what this version of you believes you can be a year from today.

- What hopes do you hold for yourself in the future around food, behavior, and lifestyle?
- What internal resources do you possess that will help you, now and always?
- What faith do you hold in your own strengths and abilities right now that you might not remember in a year?
- What message or belief about yourself did you discover this month that you never want to forget?

You have had an evolution over the past 24 days and it will continue for the rest of your life. In this moment, however, you possess a rare opportunity to write this letter. You are unhitched from a dietary habit that has been present since your first taste of sugar. This vantage point might never be available again. Don't let it slip away.

Engagement

You know what the engagement is for this day. Right now—can you decide on whether the letter is going to be pen/paper or electronic—and get to it? If it feels scary, or silly, or like something you'll do "later," I am going to invite you to step into the challenge and do it now. It doesn't even have to take more than a total of 15 minutes. Those four prompts above are just to get you rolling. If another letter all together starts forming, go with it!

I will check in with you tomorrow. Write that letter and lock it away. It's like a long-term Certificate of Deposit you are giving yourself. Yet another gift to come from this 30 Days Sugar Free.

Exit Strategies – Day 31 and Beyond

Yesterday, I was talking to you about writing that letter to your future self—gathering up the insights and takeaways from the first 24 days and using them to pop a message of strength into a time capsule that will be sent to you in a year.

If you wrote the letter—Fantastic!

If you haven't done it yet and are "thinking" about it—turn off the thinking and turn on the writing. It doesn't have to be perfect (in fact, there's no such thing!). Just connect the input of those prompts to the output of your heart and seal the deal.

Let's talk about the big white elephant in the room.

You have been brilliant with the challenge—make no mistake about that. By any measure you have hit the game-winning grand-slam of life. Right now, what's left is that courtesy run around the bases to make it official. You don't have to steal any bases, outrun a great throw by the shortstop, or worry about sliding into home.

Day 25, in most cases, is the parade down Main Street to the end. Enjoy it. Revel in it.

Options Going Forward

This is something I haven't talked about because up until today, it's been about working the challenge—finding the foods that you can eat, getting past the struggles, and looking inward for strength to keep on keeping on.

October 6 · 🌐

Today is my 150 day milestone day! I'd have never believed it possible if I hadn't actually done it myself! Thank you 30 Days Sugar Free Group! And thank you especially Barry Friedman! If it hadn't been for the fact that ▇▇▇ ▇▇▇▇ told me about the program I'd still probably be struggling with my Dr. Pepper addiction. Thank you Michele Rothstein, too, but Karl's referring me to fellow variety artist Barry really did the trick. I can't thank you or the website or this group enough. I will forever be grateful. For the newbies and the starting overs, YOU GOT THIS! WE'LL HELP!

Unlike · Comment · 👍 15 💬 9

The discussion here is about some possible options for Day 31 and beyond. I will share my experience of what each could look like. Everything in this chapter comes from watching and talking to people from various sugar free forums and communities since February, 2012.

While every person is different, I have seen some trends and I'm sharing those in hopes that they will help you find what makes sense for you moving forward.

Option 1: Continue On!

I'll jump right in and start with the best case scenario. You are on a roll. Your body doesn't know anything about time at this point and the difference between 30 days and 60 days is indistinguishable.

> *"My tastes changed so much during the 30 Days Sugar Free. When the month ended I decided to do another month. I did this three times in total and then said I'd try for the year. The truth is, there was no more trying. I was just living sugar free and it wasn't any longer about the calendar. With my experience and past relationship to food, this was my ticket out. I've never considered turning it in for a refund!"* —**Michele Rothstein, Las Vegas, NV**

Personally, I remember after my 30 Days Sugar Free that I decided to go for a year. At the end of the year, I just kept going without an end date in mind. After 30 days, I had no desire for anything containing refined or processed sugar. I remember thinking that perhaps my sweet tooth had fallen out. I was down from 36" waist pants to 32" and I had lost almost 20 lbs. There was no call to go back to eating junk, so I didn't.

My favorite analogy around sugar is this: why would I wait in line, buy a ticket, and go see a movie I didn't like the first time?

So the first option for Day 31 is to keep it looking like the past thirty days. If you do this—perfect!—and I recommend you commit to another fixed period of time. Perhaps, oh, I don't know, maybe 30 days and reevaluate at that time.

You might be called to go day to day and use your Gut Intelligence about where you are in your relationship to sugar. From what I've seen, though, this often leads to a full return to sugar within approximately two weeks.

Option 2: Dabbling in Sugar

Dabbling in sugar is the exit strategy I planned when I began the 30 Days Sugar Free challenge. I figured I'd get through the 30 days, have some new awareness, and go back to enjoying the stuff I used to love— but with a new level of maturity around it.

The thought process was something like this: I've seen the light and now I will have this super power to make sugar more like a pet fish—there to look at when I want to, but for the most part, out of sight, out of mind.

While I never got to the point of dabbling, I know many that have.

> *"For the first few days after my 30 Days Sugar Free I was laughing at sugar. How could I have ever been addicted to it? My first return was on Day 31 and I had beef jerky— of all things—that had sugar in the marinade. It tasted really strange, not at all like I remember it. The next day I had a granola bar and still felt like I was in control. I even had some ice cream that night just to show myself that I could handle it. A week later I had forgotten the challenge, put on 6 lbs., and knew that sugar had me right back where I was before I started."* **—Shelley Levine, San Diego, CA**

Shelley's case is not unusual. I have read similar stories from those that ended the challenge and decided to dabble in sugar.

I'll share another story. This one from Peter. He's one of many dabblers that have gone on and found success:

> *"I finished my 30 Days Sugar Free challenge and spent a few days in a holding pattern. Not eating any sugar but staying open to the possibility of it. Since that time (over a year now), I have been able to draw some lines in the sand that I don't cross. Nothing with high fructose corn syrup. I don't drink soda pop or eat candy. I probably would if I had the desire, it's just the thought of those things make me sick. I don't read every label either like I did during the challenge. These days I just have an intuition about what I can eat. Maybe it's that 'gut intelligence' you talked about!"* —**Peter Richmond, Austin, TX**

If your next move is to dabble, know that I support your choice 100%. You've made it this far and if the calling is to go back, you'll always have this book (and your journal!) to remind you of this time.

Option 3: This Challenge is Over—I'm Free!
There is a big part of me that salutes you for your clarity. You have done a yeoman's job of navigating the spills and chills of this 30 Days Sugar Free. It's like that time you drove all day and night to have an experience that lasted an hour. Or that time you waited in line for 24-hours to get tickets to see a rock concert. (I'm talking pre-internet here, kids!)

You had a vision and you fulfilled it. Maybe you aren't seeing the results you expected to see from the 30 Days Sugar Free (still five days to go—don't call it quits yet!) and you realize your body is just fine with your old diet.

If this is you, I truly hope you'll look back on the experience and see some positives that came from it. If nothing else, you have shown an undeniable ability to follow through. You have proved your mettle and no one can take that away.

So Why Am I Talking About this on Day 25?

Today is about planting seeds. Time goes quickly here at the end and before you know it you'll wake up on Day 31. These seeds will have had five full days to sprout, take root, and help you decide what is right for you.

You don't need to do anything with this information right now. Just reading it has started the process. The rest happens in a magically choreographed dance between your logical mind, your loving heart, and the mystery of life. The best you can do is stay out of our own way.

In Closing

A poem for whenever it feels like sugar might be the answer:

Enough

Enough. These few words are enough.
If not these words, this breath.
If not this breath, this sitting here.
This opening to the life
we have refused
again and again
until now.
Until now.

—David Whyte from: The Heart Aroused: Poetry and
the Preservation of the Soul in Corporate America

Have a powerful Day 25.

Cravings and Vigilance

On Day 21, I wrote about patterns and interrupts. I want to talk about the pattern's second cousin, the craving.

After 26 days of sugar free living, are you clear on the difference as it relates to food? Did cravings become patterns, or do patterns create cravings?

Pattern: *noun:* a reliable sample of traits, acts, tendencies, or other observable characteristics of a person, group, or institution

Craving: *noun:* an intense, urgent, or abnormal desire or longing

From a member of an online Sugar Free challenge:

> July 14 at 11:35am · 🕓
>
> So... rocky old weekend. Came within a sniff of a binge, nearly called someone to help 'stop me'... but then reminded myself that I could stop me! Two weeks now. I am eating everything that's not nailed down. But as long as it's not sugar that's ok with me. My mantra at the moment is: eating sugar won't change anything, not eating sugar will change everything 😊
>
> Unlike · Comment · 👍 16 💬 11

The distinction between pattern and craving has to do with where this person is in her journey. Go back a year and a sugar binge might very well have been a pattern. Here, with over two weeks of sugar free living under her belt, it's a flat out craving, and she dealt with it appropriately.

You see, cravings can be addressed by the left side of the brain that deals with analytical and logical thinking. You might see someone eating a piece of apple pie smothered in whipped cream and crave it. Here on Day 26, you have tools to tell yourself that a) you know what that tastes like and you're not doing that right now, b) you've only got a few days to go of this challenge and you can, if you want, have apple pie when it's over, and c) there are parts of you that feel bigger, stronger, better than ever for seeing it and not eating it. That's left brain work in action.

You've come this far and whether or not you realize it, you have a lot of pride, spirit, and strength around cravings that you didn't have a month ago. You wouldn't be here if you didn't. Without even having a camera into your life, the fact that you are here today tells me a lot about you.

Cravings are often tied to an emotional reaction. A memory, a song, a relationship, or anything else that was sweet. Your skills for change, here on Day 26, give you the latitude to make new connections. Satisfy those cravings with a perfectly ripe strawberry, some frozen banana "ice cream," or even these game-changing Chocolate Coconut Date balls which you'll find in the Member Area for Day 26. http://ILoveMeMoreThanSugar.com

You possess the ability to enjoy a healthy, sweet experience without over-indulging in something loaded with the emptiness of refined sugar. You know how to meet the call of that craving in a mindful way. The conscious selection, appreciation, and consumption of healthy sweet might very well be a new skill for you. It's one that you're ready for. Embrace it.

Essential Oils and Cravings

Several members of my online program have reported the use of essential oils in helping to curb their sugar cravings. In a ½ gallon of water, add a drop of peppermint or cinnamon essential oil. Make sure the oil is from a reputable, research-based company that uses Certified Pure Therapeutic Grade oils tested for purity such as doTerra and Native American Nutritionals.

You are Vigilant

I know some of the dark, murky creeks you have forged during the past 26 days. Being here means that you know vigilance, can recognize a craving, and know yourself well enough to deal with it. You know that there is a personal reward that will serve you for the rest of your life and that has been enough to empower you through a lot of cravings. This day is for those who have looked a cookie, pie, or soda in the eye and laughed, cried, or took a long, slow breath and walked away.

You are Grateful

Someone who makes it to this day in the challenge understands gratitude. There have been a hundred opportunities for you to eat sugar—and not one of them presented a reason good enough to get you to fold. That is a demonstration of postponed gratification which is so rare in our culture. Instead of "deserving that dessert," you have stood for deserving to not eat that dessert. Who does that?

And I'm not going to let you drop your head, kick some dirt, and say, "Shucks… anyone could do this, right?" No, your job right now, when you reach the period at the end of this sentence, is to close your eyes, take in a deep breath, put your hands over your heart, and give yourself some deep gratitude.

You are an Inspiration to Others

I know we touched on this earlier, but here on Day 26 I want to remind you that there are eyes all over you right now. Maybe you feel them, maybe not. Friends, family members, co-workers, and even those you don't know.

Recently, I took my son and his friend to the ice cream shop in town. It was almost 100 degrees outside and I wanted to surprise them with something that they'd love. They each ordered a single scoop in a cup (hey, I have my limits!), and I just watched with a smile.

A woman in her seventies was sitting with her husband and she called out to me as I walked by. She said, "I've never seen anyone buy ice cream for two kids and not get one for himself."

I was reminded about what I often say to people doing 30 Days Sugar Free—people are watching! Sugar is the most celebrated and available addiction in the world and to have control over it gets people talking. I told her that I don't eat sugar. I ate more than my share for the first 50 years of my life and it no longer had a place in my life. She asked if I missed it and what I do for relief from the heat.

I shook my water bottle and said, "Hear that? It's ice water and it makes me feel better than sugar ever did." She smiled and I wished her a great day.

It's not our job to save people from the evils of sugar. We can, however, set a grand example of possibility for those who wonder if this challenge might be right for them.

Never doubt that a small group of thoughtful, committed citizens can change the world. Indeed, it is the only thing that ever has. —Margaret Mead

Journal
Respond to these prompts in your journal:
- Three foods I used to crave
- Three foods I still crave
- What is my most compelling argument against any craving that doesn't serve me?

Engagement
While you're in the Member Area, watch a video of Constant Craving by k.d. Lang. It's a beautiful song and the lyrics offer an additional level of breadth about cravings. http://ILoveMeMoreThanSugar.com

Going Mobile – Traveling Sugar Free

How have you possibly made it to Day 27? I'm betting that four weeks ago you might have been saying, "I could never do that!" Welcome to the other side of "never."

And in case you're wondering how you got here, here's my take. You've been there every step of the way. It's been with the consciousness and focus of a monk around one of the most natural acts of humanity—eating. For each of the past 27 days, you have made some die-hard choices to do differently that which you have done in mostly the same way your entire life. Monumental change, my friend!

At this point in the challenge, many people are seeing changes including blood pressure, glucose levels, energy, surges of will power, better sleep, shifting body shape, and a loss of weight. Just as this journey has unfolded, so have the lessons and takeaways that will last far beyond the end of the month.

I didn't know what would come from putting this message out into the world, and I never imagined getting to see such interaction, connection, and transformation.

On the Road Again

There is this little piece of my life that hasn't really come up much. I briefly mentioned in this book's introduction that I am a professional juggler, but I haven't gone into exactly what that means. I want to talk about one way it relates to this 30 Days Sugar Free challenge.

It's Time For the Juggling Talk

You see, in a really, really, really small niche of the world, I'm kind of a big deal. That's right, among clowns, ventriloquists, mimes, magicians, comedians, and jugglers—I am world famous. Stay seated... here I am just another guy getting through the day without eating sugar.

What my "fame" has brought me is the coolest career in the world. As one-half of the Raspyni Brothers, I've been to just about every corner of the planet to perform my show. I have worked with the same partner since 1982, and we specialize in corporate entertainment. This includes sales meetings, trade shows, product launches, customer appreciation events, awards banquets and the like—always at the finest resorts in places like the Caribbean, Bali, Hawaii, Paris, Christchurch, and even Fargo.

I've had Elite Status on several airlines in my life and ridden in more limos than I can remember. And the backstage treats—oh my—50 Shades of Sugar that always call with a sweet whisper to "just try one."

Yes, I've had hundreds of opportunities to violate my gluten and sugar free life—and they don't stop. Temptation happens outside of the home and that's a part of our work here in this challenge. What to do "out there"?

Preparation and Standing in the Fire

The linchpins of success in a sugar free challenge, as you know, are preparation and being able to stand strong in the face of temptation.

I don't dare go on the road without enough sugar free food to keep me clear of anything available at airports. Take away the sugar and gluten at an airport and what remains is a big building, some connected chairs, and a lot of over-priced bottles of water. Meat is marinated in a sugary concoction. Nuts are covered in sweetened chocolate. Dried fruit is sprayed with enough chemicals to keep it pretty and often has added sugar. There is no oasis for the health conscious traveler in this world. Well, there is always the Wolfgang Puck $12.99 iceberg salad with oil/vinegar, if you can find it. Yum!

Here's My Sugar Free (and Gluten Free) Travel Pack:
- Organic Corn Thins by Real Foods
- Beef Jerky – Homemade (Organic grass-fed tri-tip marinated in

ginger, garlic, tamari sauce, then dehydrated for 8 hours)
- Fruit – Fuji apples, plums, Asian pears, dried mango, box or two of raisins – all travel well and give good energy and fiber
- Water – Tons of it. I fill my bottle (after dumping it to keep the plane safe!) at a drinking fountain. Many airports now have water filling stations, which is cold and presumably filtered.
- Tuna Packets – Great protein and easy to pack. Delicious on the Corn Thins. Grab a mustard pack from one of the airport counters.
- Veggies – Celery and carrots are sturdy in a zip-lock bag. Cut red peppers are a special treat that don't last all that long.
- Almond butter packets—Protein without any mess or fuss. Yummy on the aforementioned Corn Thins, too.
- String cheese – They last quite a while in those peel packets.
- Trail mix—My own concoction of favorite nuts, coconut flakes, and dried fruit.

There are the basics. On the road I do menu research as previously mentioned. For the most part, I eat fish, chicken with rice, and salad with no sauces. For dessert, I'm the guy who orders herbal tea.

When possible, I hit Whole Foods or a local food co-op and do a massive salad bar. Game changing. Cashiers look at me with confusion and families move out of the way when they see my tongs reaching. It's my reward to myself for standing strong in my commitment to myself and my family.

If you're in one place for a few days, always ask for a mini fridge and stock up.

The road has become a lot less about the food over the years—and more about the experience; staying centered in the confusion and crowds; taking care of myself; and watching the ordinary citizens line up for Big Macs and frozen yogurt. People watching is a powerful motivator for a sugar free life.

Journal

Write your favorite food travel ideas in your journal—either from the above list or your own ideas. Then when you go on a trip, you'll have a handy list.

Engagement

Well, how could I talk about my life without offering a video sample. This really has nothing to do with sugar free—but it is good for some laughs and there's nothing wrong with that. Find the video of my performance at a TED Conference in the Member Area Resources for Day 27. http://ILoveMeMoreThanSugar.com

The sugar offerings at a TED Conference are legendary. My 6th TED appearance was in March, 2014 and it was my first one sugar free. No problem! The attendees and other speakers were sweet enough for me.

Day 27 of choosing not to eat sugar... how beautiful is that?

How I See You Now

Twenty eight days down—did you ever imagine you'd be here? Seriously... if you could go back in time three months and a fortune teller looked into a crystal ball and told you that soon you would be almost finished with 30 Days Sugar Free, would you have believed her?

It's both a coincidence and a truckload of hard work that has brought you to this place in life. I hope you are taking a moment to breathe in the magic of mystery and the reward of dedication. Both are spectacular gifts.

Earlier, I talked about the moment of decision to do this challenge and I want you to wrap your brain around the reality. It's your work—minute by minute—that has gotten you here. Beyond the sugar, I want you to know that this power of change is available to you for anything you want to achieve in your life. You have made the change with arguably the most difficult situation and substance in the free world—addiction and sugar.

After climbing that hill—what's the next challenge? New job? Write a book? Run a 10K? You overcame something harder than any of these in the first 10 days of this challenge. You broke a habit, one that involved social pressure, chemical addiction, taste buds, comfort, neurological programming, and the short-term convenience of eating whatever you want.

You have what it takes to make big changes. You've done what it takes and you might even have surprised yourself. Don't you dare skip the step where you acknowledge yourself for this gift. Walk through the downtown area of where you live. See all those people? Zero of them have done what you have done in the last four weeks.

If I sound excited, it's because I am. I've seen so many people want this, try this, dabble in this—everything except finish it. I've heard stories of why they can't and they all just sound like that little tune that plays in cartoons when something goes wrong—Waaa Waaa Waaa— wwwaaaa!

Do it or don't. You are doing it.

Spoonful of Sugar Free — Interview with Alex!

I told you she was coming! Visit the Member Area for Day 28 and you'll find an exclusive interview. I hope you can listen to it today. It's an intelligent and insightful conversation with Alex Curtis of SpoonfulOfSugarFree.com!

As you'll hear from this bright and engaging 20-something, she's been sugar free since age 13 and has given the world so many wonderful ideas about desserts, meals, and healthy living. She's a rock star athlete—competitive tennis player—and truly taking life by the horns and giving it a ride.

What I love so much about Alex's cooking is that she stays away from any sort of alternative sweetener—no stevia, agave, or any of the "... ose" sweeteners. She's a beaming manifestation of the possibility.

"Once you just do it—break that bond with sugar
—you don't crave it anymore. You don't have that need to
eat it." —Alex Curtis of SpoonfulOfSugarFree.com

Find her interview in the Member Area.
http://ILoveMeMoreThanSugar.com

Journal

Alex started her sugar free journey at the age of 13. What if you could influence a young person to perhaps think and act differently about their food choices? Can you pick one young person with whom you'd be willing to share your experience so far? Write the key points you would like to highlight in that conversation.

Engagement

In the interview, Alex mentions her Flourless Chocolate Cake. This might be the single best invention since the airplane.

I suggest you plan out the ingredients, plan ahead for a special date (like maybe in two days when the 30 Days Sugar Free challenge ends?!?), and bake this bad boy to golden perfection.

DAY 29

Accountability Drives Action

On Day 25, we talked about what Day 31 could look like. That seed has had four days to take root and here on Day 29, I'm guessing that you have a pretty good idea of what you're doing on Day 31. If that's the case, then congratulations. Now let's see what we can do to make sure that sticks.

I use accountability in my businesses and personal life. I want to invite you to use it to move forward from this challenge.

This book is in existence because I set it as a goal and then was held accountable for each step of the creation.

Accountability is easy. It takes very little time and I'll share a protocol I use to keep it simple.

Accountability Groups

Find someone and create an accountability group. Even better—find two others! These groups work really well with three people.

To start, think about two other people you would like to invite. It's important that the group isn't with two other people that you have known your whole life. For this process to be truly supportive, it should be with people you don't know all that well.

Try to work with people you admire and respect. Raise your game by engaging with people who are at or above your level of dedication. Reach out. Make the difficult call. Someone might be waiting for this exact invitation.

Find a time to meet on the phone/Skype/Google Hangout or in person. During that first meeting, you are going to brainstorm around your goals. Each of you will set a S.M.A.R.T. goal—something just outside of your comfort zone. This could be about a creative idea, a work vision, or even about your relationship moving forward with sugar. Remember the S.M.A.R.T. goals?

Specific – Is it clear, without ambiguity?
Measurable – Is there a number in it?
Achievable – Is there an action-oriented verb, for example, lose, complete, or weigh?
Relevant – Is the goal consistent with your expectations?
Time Bound – Is there a specific date or time you'll be complete?

At the end of the brainstorming session, you are going to make a commitment. Each person in the group does their own brainstorming and commitment. When you meet next (at least once a week to get going), each person is asked four questions regarding their experience and fulfillment of their commitment.

The Four Questions

What was your commitment? Simply restate your entire commitment as you originally said it.

Did you do it? This is a straight yes or no. Not a time for excuses or story—it's really clean and easy—yes or no.

What did you choose to do instead? We have become masters of choice over these 29 days. Every moment we get to choose and that realization has given us a lot of personal power. Question 3 is about owning that power and being clear about what you choose to do instead.

Where else does this show up in your life? This question is a chance for the person doing the accountability to look at how else this might show up in their life. Are you often late? Do you regularly say you are going to do something and then not do it?

If there is an admission/realization—don't try to fix the person. Let them have that realization and decide for themselves what they want to do moving forward.

How you do anything is how you do everything—and these accountability groups can uncover holes that have cost you lots of money and time over the years. These groups aren't about guilt or shame. They are all about helping you keep your word so that you can get what you wanted when you made the commitment.

Let's recap the format after you have your group and are ready to meet:
- Brainstorm
- Set S.M.A.R.T. goals
- Make a commitment
- Four Questions

That's the long and short of accountability. Take these steps and get set for moving forward with a conscious plan (for sugar and/or your life) once this challenge ends. Get someone to hear it and hold you accountable.

Rise up. This is your time to play your biggest game.

DAY 30
Cliff Notes and the Celebration

What a long strange trip it's been. What started with you picking up this book has led you into a mysterious 30-day adventure that I doubt you'll ever forget. Today is the caboose of the challenge; the final day of the original agreement you made with yourself on Day 1. Dozens or hundreds of conscious choices later, you are at the day that probably seemed unimaginable.

I have been exactly where you are and I remember how good it felt. I hope you are in similar states of buzz, power, and self-confidence. And just as it makes no sense to try and give your child life advice when you drop her off at the college dorm room, I won't spend today handing you new ways to think or interact with sugar. There has been plenty of that in the last 30 days and you have come so far from where you started.

How About a Real Simple Takeaway?
You have found a new side of yourself through this challenge. I have no doubt people will come and ask you what they can do to eat healthier or how they can help their children have a healthier relationship with food. You'll have an opportunity to inspire and inform.

While very few people will do the dedicated 30 day challenge that you are finishing today, here is a simple 4-step guideline you can offer. This comes via Doctor Robert Lustig's talk called *Sugar: The Bitter Truth*.

1. Get rid of every sugared liquid in the house. Bar none. Only water, milk, unsweetened iced tea, unsweetened coffee. There is no such thing as a good sugar beverage. Period.
2. Eat your carbohydrates with fiber. Why? Because fiber is good for you.
3. Wait 20 minutes for second portions. Give your body time to tell you that it's full!
4. Finally, and this is for your kids, have them buy their screen time minute for minute with physical activity. That's the hardest one to do. If you play for ½ hour, you can watch TV for ½ hour. You want to watch TV for an hour? Play for an hour.

Doctor Lustig offers this simple recipe to the parents of his pediatric patients who are overweight, obese, lethargic, and unmotivated. He follows up with his patients every three months. He asks them, "Is it working?" What do you think he hears in reply? "Yeah, it's working!"

Two Requests

First – Keep this book handy for a while. As you transition back to life after the challenge, you might want to reference your journal entries, find a passage that impacted you, or even go through it again. I've had people write to me after the challenge and tell me that they really fell apart. (See the Dabbler's Guide in the next chapter.) By having the book in your immediate vicinity, you'll be visually reminded of what you have accomplished. Second—Celebrate! You've earned it and it's time to share it proudly. Your 30 Days Sugar Free badge is available in the Member Area. http://ILoveMeMoreThanSugar.com

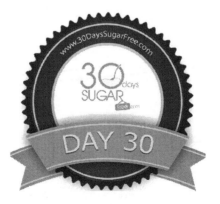

So many people do this challenge because they see that a friend has lived (and thrived) through it. What a huge gift to them—one that can forever change their life.

Know that regardless of the path you choose with your relationship to sugar, I couldn't be more proud of where you are standing right here, right now.

Birdwings

Your grief for what you've
lost lifts a mirror up to where
you're bravely working.
Expecting the worst, you look,
and instead, here's the joyful face
you've been wanting to see.
Your hand opens and closes
and opens and closes.
If it were always a fist
or always stretched open,
you would be paralyzed.
Your deepest presence
is in every small contracting and expanding,
the two as beautifully balanced and coordinated
as bird wings.
—Rumi

Dabbler's Guide

The toughest part of writing this chapter is the possibility that it might look like I am encouraging you to get back into eating processed sugar.

Group
October 1 · New Iberia, LA · 🖼

Today I have been sugar free for ONE WHOLE YEAR! This program has truly changed my life. I will be forever grateful to Barry & Michell for sharing their knowledge with me. I went from a size 16 to a size 4. I have struggled with my weight and addiction to sugar most of my life. I am now free from the bondage that food had on me. I never want to go back.

Like · Comment · 👍 24 💬 17

Let me be clear up front—I believe that if you have made it through the 30 Days Sugar Free, you are an over-the-top Super Hero. Your picture should be in *Ripley's Believe It or Not*. Local Health Departments should be inviting you to stand at the entrance to the food court at the county fair and tell people there's a better way. You should be certified to speak to groups and lead movements.

You've done the hard part and going back into sugar is a slippery slope. I haven't dared re-entry so, clearly, I am biased. I have no solid research to share in this chapter. I am going to settle for talking about what I believe could work, and mention some of the results others have had after their 30 Days Sugar Free. In Day 25, I spoke about the options going forward after the challenge. You can review those if you haven't already made up your mind. In a nutshell, they are:

1. Set another achievable goal and hit it (say... 30 days?)
2. Be a Dabbler
3. I'm Done – Going Back to Sugar.

This chapter will address the second option, because the other two are pretty clear!

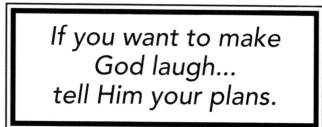

If you want to make God laugh... tell Him your plans.

The Dabbler

I am going to break The Dabbler into two camps—*The Occasional* and *The Better Than I Was Before*.

While both of the groups are built on a foundation of good intention, the tricky part is that neither of them have the support beams you leaned on for your 30 day challenge: abstinence and accountability.

In the absence of these two pillars, there is a huge possibility of old ways moving back in and taking over control of the bus.

Think lottery winners—70% are broke within two years of winning and another 15% aren't far behind.

Now, the last thing we want to do is compare you to a lottery winner. What you have done has left you feeling better, looking better, sleeping better, living better—but unlike a lottery winner, you have worked for every single bit of it. You've faced demons and battled off temptation.

The lottery winners walked into a market and plunked down a dollar.

Both of you, however, are at a moment that few other people on the planet will ever experience—a change that touches every single moment of life as you know it. The version of you that ruled the day before this 30 day challenge still lives inside. His or her dream, now that the challenge is over, is that sugar will return so things can get back to normal.

That's where the slippery part begins.

You've witnessed the power of your systems ganging up and fighting for what they want. Remember those early days of the challenge—dreams, shakes, emotions running high, and the ever-popular cravings that assured you that they'd be satiated and move on if you'd just feed them a little bit? But you didn't. You refused to give in. Maybe it was your commitment. Maybe it was your support team. Whatever you want to call it, the outcome was that you chose to love yourself more than sugar.

The Occasional Dabbler

Just as you had a plan for your 30 Days Sugar Free, I recommend you give yourself a couple of railings to keep you balanced over the next 30 days.

Breakfast – Stick to a high protein morning. This will continue to serve you by setting that solid, non-sweet foundation for your entire day. I can't, in good faith, recommend anything sugar sweetened for the morning meal. Even if you are committed to bringing processed sugar back into your diet, please don't do it at breakfast. Make this singular change the one that sticks.

Lunch – This is probably the best time to introduce sugar (oh, this is hard to write!) if that's the way you're going. Your protein level has been set with a good breakfast and you'll have a lot of hours for your body to work it out before bed.

For the first week, stick to cleaner sugars such as maple syrup—a little goes a very long way. Local, organic honey is also very versatile as a sweetener. Your system is so clean right now, don't even think of jumping back to where you used to be. A bag of M&Ms at this point could be hazardous to your health in a lot of ways.

Dinner – Ease into the evening with a meal that will support your system. Night is the time for sleep, renewal, and purification. The organs work during this down period and the easier you can make it on them, the easier they'll make it on you. Keep desserts simple - a small cookie, a small scoop of ice cream. Remember that food's role is to fuel the body, not to blanket emotions.

Snacks – Here's where, if you're not careful, you can head south faster than a van full of Texas A&M students on Spring Break. Over the past 30 days, perhaps more than any other category of eating, you have refined your habits around snacking. Opening the flood gates here can easily turn into the eye of the storm.

So what do I recommend for The Occasional Dabbler when it comes to snack time?

- First – make sure you're actually hungry. Is this something that can be satisfied with 16 ounces of water? Constant snacking is the oil on this slippery slope back to a life of sugar.
- If you are hungry, and want something sweet:
  — Eat it and then drink plenty of water... keep it moving.
  — Don't overeat. That fourth Reese's Peanut Butter Cup tastes the exact same as the first three.
- Don't let the sugar go into a shadow or shameful place. You might want to check in with someone who supported you through the challenge and just let them know what's up.
- Take note on how you feel afterward: physically, mentally, emotionally, internally. You'd be a gift to a University's research department on that first bite of a candy bar after 30 Days Sugar Free! As you witnessed over the past 30 days, what you eat really does define how you feel, look, interact, sleep, and think.

It's probably painfully obvious that I'm not very excited about you going back to sugar. The truth is that I've seen it go bad, even with the best intentions.

You've come this far. Probably the most important thing you can do here on your 31st day is to take inventory of who you are, at this moment, from this sugar free place, and consciously decide where you want to go from here.

Believe it or not, this is a view you might never have again.

The "Better Than I Was Before Dabbler"

You know who you are! You white-knuckled the last 30 days and by hook or by crook, you made it through. You have no intention of setting a new goal and continuing on.

First off—let me say this—I am proud of you! Heck, I envy you. Your clarity sets you up for success because you aren't making any clear commitment. Your devil-may-care attitude makes you fail proof.

Understand one thing—and know it in your heart. You are always welcome to come back. Many left the challenge with the intent of being *better than I was before* and got pulled into the wreckage.

> *"No, not going strong. Not only did I fall off the wagon, but it rolled over me and I'm mangled beyond belief. This whole trying to get healthy, making good choices, etc. has been difficult. I'm trying really hard to scrape myself off the sidewalk and get back with the program. I really, really need to catch this now instead of letting too much more time pass by. I keep telling myself, 'You did it. You did it for a whole 30 days! You can do this!' But I'm having a hard time convincing myself, I guess.*
>
> *I think the biggest advice I would give anyone is... DON'T dabble in old, bad habits. Just let them go. It feels SO great to be achieving such a noble goal while in the midst of the 30 days, but if you then think you can have sugar 'once in a while,' or just a bit of this or that once the 30 days is done, well, you are setting yourself up for some bad times. I really thought I could be 'mostly' sugar free and then get right back with it, but that isn't what happened. I feel SO good when making better nutritional choices, i.e. sugar free. I'm mad and sad and disgusted with myself for slipping back into habits that are literally killing me.*
>
> *However, I have not given up hope and I am putting things into place to be able to get back with it SOON, as in a day or two at most. I'm also working through some things with a good therapist to try to get to the bottom of my eating habits... I certainly don't eat because I'm*

hungry or choose the bad stuff because I really like it... it's
so weird how I can eat 'crap' that I really don't even care
for, but I feel compelled to eat it. I can tell you that I have
a lot more compassion for alcoholics. It's rough having
something inanimate have such control over me. Yuck."
—An Alumni of 30 Days Sugar Free

It's not my style to paint messy pictures. I tend to hover on the side of "radically inspirational and supportive." In that same spirit, I will stay here and hold the place together if you step away. Come back, whenever you want, no excuses necessary.

I regularly hear from alumni about how they wish they had stayed on and hope to come back. Never have I gotten an email that says, "I went back to how I was before and I've never been so happy—you are leading a group of nut jobs!"

An Afterword

Writing this book required me to slay a number of dragons that live in my mind. Each of them came along at various times, checked in under pseudo names, and carried a promise of keeping me safe.

One told me that I should just stop because I'm not a doctor and what I have to say doesn't matter. Another promised me that I was special for removing sugar from my life and no one else who will buy this book could ever do it—and I should just stop writing it. A third actually had control of my head and would occasionally turn me around in my office, scan the walls, and say, "I don't see a diploma in Sugar Free Coaching, do you?"

I am not alone. I have sat in enough group counseling sessions, workshops, classes, and retreats to know that the biggest battles we fight are the ones going on inside. The shiny object, new app, or viral video that wants to keep us away from doing our work and changing the world will always be there.

As I write the final page of this book, I draw my razor-sharp sword and take another clean and meaningful slice at all those collective voices. I also thank them, because part of me wonders if I would even be here without them.

You and I just completed a journey together and I want to thank you for believing in yourself. I'm honored, humbled, and here to support you moving forward.

Because I have setup an online Member Area for this book, we have the remarkable opportunity to stay in touch and encourage one another. For as long as it serves you, I hope you'll take advantage of everything available in that portal.

Barry Friedman
The Foothills of the Sierra Mountains, CA
November 30, 2014

50+ Names for Sugar

Names for Sugar You Can Eat

Raw Organic Honey (1/4 cup over the month)
Lactose (naturally occurring in milk)
Fruit
Fruit Juice without added sweeteners

50+ Names for Sugar

Agave

Amino Sweet

Aspartame

Barley malt

Beet sugar

Brown sugar

Buttered syrup

Cane juice

Cane juice crystals

Cane sugar

Caramel

Corn syrup

Corn syrup solids

Confectioner's sugar

Carob syrup

Castor sugar

Date sugar

Demerara sugar

Dextran

Dextrose

Diastatic malt

Diatase

Ethyl maltol

Evaporated cane juice

Fructose

Fruit juice

Fruit juice concentrate

Galactose

Glucose

Glucose solids

Golden sugar
Golden syrup
Grape sugar
High-fructose corn syrup
Honey
Icing sugar
Invert sugar
Lactose
Maltodextrin
Maltose
Malt syrup
Maple syrup
Molasses

Muscovado sugar
Panocha
Raw sugar
Refiner's syrup
Rice syrup
Sorbitol
Sorghum syrup
Sucrose
Sugar
Treacle
Turbinado sugar
Yellow sugar

Shopping List

Here are items that you can safely eat during your 30 Days Sugar Free. There is no need to start at the top and buy everything—it's not that kind of list!

Legumes and Beans

Use these to spice up soups, add protein to dishes, and create simple snacks. There are many more and these are the ones I recommend for getting started.

Adzuki beans

Black beans

Black-eyed peas

Broad beans

Butter beans

Chickpeas

Fava beans

Garbanzo beans

Great northern beans

Kidney beans

Lentils

Lima beans

Miso

Moth beans

Okra

Peas

Peanuts

Red beans

Refried beans

Rice beans

Soybeans (edamame)

Split peas

Tempeh

Tofu

White beans

Yellow beans

Dairy

These products will list some sugar on the Nutrition Facts label. This is naturally occurring in the lactose. Always check the ingredients and avoid any that list a form of added sugar/sweetener.

NOTE: Watch out when buying shredded cheese. You'll see dextrose on the list of ingredients. Shredding cheese is not that hard!

Blue cheese	Gouda cheese
Brie	Milk
Butter	Monterey Jack cheese
Buttermilk	Mozzarella cheese
Cheddar cheese	Muenster cheese
Colby cheese	Parmesan cheese
Cream cheese	Provolone cheese
Cottage cheese	Ricotta cheese
Feta cheese	Romano cheese
Goat cheese	Swiss cheese
Goat yogurt	Yogurt (plain – ingredients: milk & probiotics only)

Meat/Poultry

Check labels for all dried and cured meats. Often sugar is used during these processes.

Beef	Pheasant
Bison	Pork
Buffalo	Pot Roast
Chicken	Quail
Duck	Sirloin
Eggs	Steaks
Frogs Legs	Tenderloin
Goose	Turkey
Lamb	Faux Meat brands w/o sugar
Liver	

Nuts and Seeds

Confirm that the nut butters you buy have no added sugar.

Almond butter
Almonds
Cashew butter
Cashews
Hazelnuts
Hickory nuts
Lotus seeds
Macadamia nuts
Peanut butter

Peanuts
Pecans
Pistachios
Pumpkin seeds
Sesame seeds
Soy nut butter
Soy nuts
Tahini (or Sesame butter)
Walnuts

Seafood

Abalone Tuna
Anchovy
Bass
Carp
Catfish
Caviar
Clams
Cod
Crab
Eel
Flounder
Grouper
Haddock
Halibut
Herring
Kingfish
Lobster
Mackerel
Mussels, blue

Octopus
Orange roughy
Oysters
Salmon
Sardines, canned in water
Scallops
Sea bass
Sea trout
Shrimp
Smelt
Snapper
Squid
Sturgeon
Swordfish
Trout
Tuna, canned in water
Whitefish
Yellow tail

Fruit

Apples
Apricots
Asian pears
Avocados
Bananas
Blackberries
Blueberries
Boysenberries
Cantaloupe
Carambola
Casaba melon
Cherries
Crabapples
Cranberries
Durian
Figs
Grapefruit
Grapes

Guava
Honeydew melon
Kiwi
Kumquats
Lemon
Lime
Mango
Nectarine
Orange
Papaya
Passion fruit
Peach
Pear
Pineapple
Plum
Raspberries
Strawberries
Tangerine

Vegetables

Alfalfa sprouts
Artichoke
Arugula
Asparagus
Bamboo shoots
Bean Sprouts
Beets
Bok Choy
Broccoli
Brussels sprouts
Cabbage
Carrot
Cauliflower
Celery
Cucumber
Eggplant
Fennel
Garden cress
Gourd
Green beans
Jicama
Kale
Leeks
Lettuce, many varieties!

Mushrooms
Mustard greens
Okra
Onions
Parsnip
Peppers
Pumpkin
Radicchio
Radish
Rhubarb
Rutabaga
Scallions
Seaweed
Snap peas
Spinach
Squash, many varieties
Swiss chard
Tomatoes
Turnip
Water chestnuts
Watercress
Yam/Sweet potatoes
Zucchini

Toppings and Oils

Bragg Liquid Aminos

Coconut oil (good for high heat)

Flax oil supplement (do not heat)

Olive oil

Almond oil

Sesame oil

Butter

Ghee (clarified butter)

Lemon juice

Mustard

Olives

Pickles

Roasted pepper

Mayonnaise – sugar free (Trader Joe's and Ojai Cook brands)

Tabasco Sauce

Trader Joe's Goddess or Newman's Goddess Dressing

Vinegars – Apple cider, Balsamic

Breads

Check labels carefully—these brands have reportedly had sugar free offerings in their product line.

Dave's Killer Bread

The Baker

Damascus Bakeries

Food for Life

French Meadow

Genuine Bavarian

Manna Breads

Puebla Foods

Real Foods Organic Corn Thins

Stickling's

Sunnyvale Bakery

Whole Foods

Breakfast Cereal

Arrowhead Mills Puffed Corn

Barbara's Bakery Original Shredded Wheat

Puffed Kashi, Seven Whole Grains & Sesame

Cooked Cereals

Bob's Red Mill Mighty Tasty Hot Cereal

Kashi Pilaf

Old Wessex Ltd. 100% natural whole grain Scottish Chewy Porridge Oats

McCann's Steel Cut Irish Oatmeal

Arrowhead Mills 7-Grain Cereal

Crackers

Amy Lyn's Original Flax Thins

Hol-Grain Brown Rice Crackers

Conrad Rice Mill Brown Rice with a Touch of Salt

Cracker Flax, Tomato Onion

Finn Crisps

Glaser Farms

Kavli (5-Grain, Hearty Thick, Hearty Rye, All Natural Crispy Thin)

Lydia's Lovin' Foods Italian Crackers

Ryvita

Scandinavian Bran Crispbread

365 Baked Woven Wheats

Wasa Original Crispbread Light Rye

Yehuda Organic Matzo

Luke's Organic Crackers

Salad Dressings

Annie's Naturals Dressings

Cindy's Kitchen Rosemary & Roasted Garlic Vinaigrette

Drew's All Natural Dressings

Whole Foods Italian Vinaigrette

Stonewall Kitchen Roasted Red Pepper Vinaigrette

Hot Dogs

Applegate Farms Natural Uncured Turkey Hot Dogs

Bilinski's All Natural Gourmet Chicken Sausage, Sun-Dried Tomato and Basil or Spinach-Garlic & Fennel

Hans' All Natural Chicken Sausage, Sun-Dried Tomato and Fresh Basil

Salsa
Check your store for fresh salsa with no added sugar

Acknowledgements

It is said that a kitchen remodel is the #1 event that can ruin a marriage. I'm guessing that writing a book comes in a close second. The idea for this project came to me like so many others—during a mountain bike ride—and that was the first and only part of it I accomplished alone.

To Annie Keeling Friedman, my wife since 1987, who has worn many different hats in conjunction with this project: sugar free partner, writing coach/editor (I totally piggy backed off that MFA in Creative Writing of yours!), moral support champion, meal deliverer to my office, and whip slinger when resistance took hold. This would never have seen the light of day without you. Thank you for believing in me.

To my son, Zed. You, dear boy, were standing right across from me on Leap Day 2012 when I first spoke about doing a single day sugar free. You lost out on a lot of trampoline bouncing, unicycle rides, video-making, mountain biking, and laughs over the past 9 months. I'm ready to jump back into all of that and more now that this book is baked to a golden brown. Also, as the only person in our house that eats sugar, I'm glad you are seeing another possibility—just in case you ever want to give it a go!

Daniel Holzman has been the other half of my 'real job' since 1982. The journeys of the Raspyni Brothers would make a great book—and just might one day. In the meantime, I want to let you know that your friendship and creativity have been important ingredients in my life. Who books that gig?

I'm a part of two mastermind groups who have stood by me during the entire journey. Brian McGovern, Jeff and Stephanie Padovani, Matthew Blom, Jacob Griscom, Christian & Sonika Pedersen, Jai Dev Singh—you each have added so much to my life. Thank you for showing up, week after week, to reflect back what you hear, and offer what you believe.

Several coaches have inspired me to reach higher (much higher, in fact) than I originally planned. Machen McDonald, Ray Arata, and Clint Arthur each provided unique approaches to the art of coaching and are model representatives of the profession. Thanks to each of you for being strong enough to coach from the heart.

In February of 2008, I showed up for a Men's Training Weekend put on by The ManKind Project. There isn't a cell of my being that has been the same since that day. Measuring the value of what that organization has shown me about living a life of integrity and authenticity would be impossible. Thank you to all my brothers who are doing their work to make this a better world.

Finally, to you, the reader of this book. We are kindred spirits and my hope is that one day we'll meet, virtually or in real life. The time we have spent together during this book gives me hope for the human race. We are always able to create a new reality and you, my friend, are living proof.

Photo Credits

All photos were originally created or owned by the subject unless otherwise noted below. Those photos not attributed were purchased by the author.

Sugar Loaf: By Petr Adam Dohnálek (Own work) [CC-BY-SA-3.0-cz (http://creativecommons.org/licenses/by-sa/3.0/cz/deed.en)], via Wikimedia Commons

Arlene Krantz: Photo by Julie Hopkins, www.CameraCreations.net

Live in the na'au: Tony Bonnici

Pg 220 – Courtesy of DAVID Magazine, Photo: Steve Wilson

Made in the USA
Charleston, SC
10 November 2015